Se_____ 19 1982

To Maggie and Norman.

affectionately,

Helen

Neil, Leni and Daniel Peter
with love

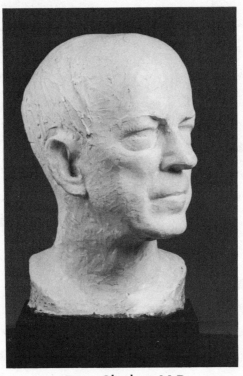

By Oscar Nemon

I. Peter Glauber, M.D.
1899-1966

Practicing psychoanalyst in New York City and Westchester; chief of Lenox Hill Psychiatric Clinic; attending psychiatrist at the Hillside Hospital; consultant to the Child Guidance Clinic of the Jewish Board of Guardians in New York; Jewish Community Services of Westchester; Children's Village in Dobbs Ferry; Hawthorne Cedar Knolls School; Associated Therapists of Westchester; director of a private treatment service for functional speech disorders. Fellow of the New York Academy of Medicine and the American Psychiatric Association; Diplomate of the American Board of Psychiatry and Neurology; member of the New York Psychoanalytic Society and the American Psychoanalytic Association. President of the Westchester Psychoanalytic Society (1963); instructor in Psychiatry at the New York University College of Medicine and a Supervisor in Psychotherapy, the New York Psychoanalytic Institute Treatment Center.

aggression as is the case in patients with stuttering. Mahler stated that patients with tics often exhibit clonic stammering but almost never tonic.

On the centennial occasion of Freud's birth, Dr. Glauber presented his paper, "Freud's Contributions on Stuttering: Their Relation to Some Current Insights," at a meeting of the New York Psychoanalytic Society, October 16, 1956.

Dr. Smiley Blanton opened the discussion: "I became interested in stuttering more than fifty years ago. There's been great progress from that time to this in the understanding of stuttering. In those days when I began, it was said to be due to some difficulty with the breathing, but I found, in analyzing a good many cases of stuttering, that the condition, at least in the cases I had, four or five, that it was more of an anal fixation which is a transference over to the oral area . . . I had the opportunity of working with Dr. Freud for more than a year, and one day I asked him if I might spend a little time telling him what my theory of stuttering was. He shrugged his shoulders as if to say—well, if you want to, you can, but he would much rather do something else. So I spent about twenty minutes giving him generally the idea I am now giving you, and he replied: 'I know very little about stuttering. I never analyzed a stutterer. You may well be right,' he said, 'but I'm sure there must be some organic factor.' And I said, 'Do you mean by organic factor the fact that the speech area is not properly fixed on one side, that is, the opposite preferential hand?' He said: 'I don't know, but I think there's some organic factor.' I said: 'Do you mean some weakness of the mechanism of speech?' And he shrugged and made a sound in his throat as if to say: 'I don't know, and let's say no more about it.' So that was what Freud had to say about stuttering to me when I was back there one summer in 1935. Dr. Glauber has gone more deeply into the analysis of the stutterer than anyone else I know, and I think he has made a real contribution to the subject. I think we all should be grateful to him."

Dr. Bernard Meyer stated, "On several counts we are indebted to Dr. Glauber for his presentation of this evening's interesting and stimulating paper. The subject of stuttering continues to evoke widespread interest and speculations and it has probably engaged

Dr. Melitta Sperling: "What I wanted really to speak about is my gratitude that Dr. Glauber by his presentation confirmed some of the findings which I have made in the treatment of children with psychosomatic disorders; three of whom were stuttering children. I found it was a specific relationship between mother and child which was an important basic factor in the etiology and in the dynamics of the child's illness. Mother and child function as a psychological unit as it were . . . ."

Dr. Bernard Meyer: "My own experience in analysis of stutterers is quite comparable to what has been described by Dr. Glauber. I have had no experience in the analysis of mothers of stutterers, aside from what I have heard through the patients. In keeping with his remarks about identification, I came upon one mother who, every night before she put her little boy to bed, used to wet his hair and comb it very neatly, and then tucked him into bed. This was done in the event that visitors might come to the house and want to see what her child looked like while he was asleep . . . to be sure that he would make a nice impression . . . ."

Dr. Margaret Ribble, in the discussion of Dr. Glauber's presentation, "Ego Development and the Character of the Stutterer," * May 10, 1949, observed two types of phallic mothers. The first type experienced delivery as a castration and rejected the infant as soon as it was born. The second type treated the infant as a material phallus as long as it was tiny and helpless but rejected the child when it began to walk and talk, i.e., to become independent. Ribble speculated that rejection at this stage in the infant's development might well result in stuttering.

Dr. Margaret S. Mahler compared her conclusions about patients with tics with those of Dr. Glauber about stutterers and commented that in both there is a pathological mother-child relationship and both have fixations at a very early narcissistic level. However, in patients with tics the primary conflicts as well as the symptoms concern muscular, phallic aggression, rather than oral

---

*Dr. Charles Brenner abstracted Dr. Glauber's paper and the discussion for the *Notes* section of the *Psychoanalytic Quarterly*, 19, 1950, No. 1.

Comments by Dr. Glauber's Colleagues on Some of the Papers Presented in This Collection

At the New York Psychoanalytic Society meeting at which Dr. Glauber's paper on "The Mother in the Etiology of Stuttering" was presented, discussants made the following comments:

Dr. Bertram Lewin: "I wonder how many of you have the same feeling as I have in hearing such a remarkable paper devoted to stuttering. . . . Dr. Glauber has made one extremely interesting contribution, not only to stuttering, . . . this had been a study of motherhood, and of preoedipal or pre-genital motherhood . . . I am extremely grateful to Dr. Glauber for his wealth of material and richness of interpretation. I found many of his formulations very striking. For example, that the stuttering speaker had been a stuttering eater before he spoke."

Dr. Phyllis Greenacre: "Dr. Glauber's presentation of the personality of the mother as being the nuclear cause of the stuttering of the son, . . . four to one times as frequently as of the daughter. He sees the problem, essentially as that of a woman never separated from, really, and appersonated by her mother, who has grave problems in her marriage, because of her effort to reproduce this state, and especially in her relation to her children with whom she actually does repeat the process. He believes that this separation problem with its deep, passive desire for union and counteracting separation aggression and anxiety permeates the whole personality of the mother and is passed on by her to her sons more frequently than to her daughters. This conception seems to me an important contribution."

classical neuroses make use of this fixation in the automatism. This fixation determines a special type of superimposed character disorder which in general reflects the structure of the symptom. The symptom, and in part the character, cannot be explicated in terms of the classical neurotic symptom. Rather it can be in special terms—that of a trauma affecting an automatism producing a fixation on it and on its defense. . . .

"Classical psychoanalytic technique may succeed in resolving the neurotic elements. *Successful treatment of the primary fixation requires reeducational methods.*"

This volume has been organized so as to reflect the interaction of Dr. Glauber's varied interests. Part I contains a psychoanalytic view of stuttering—its dynamics, its treatment, and a review of the literature on the subject. In order to present Dr. Glauber's views on stuttering in as systematic a way as possible, Part I—except for Chapter 3, "Freud's Contributions on Stuttering: Their Relation to Some Current Insights;" and Chapter 6, "Projective Tests in the Treatment of Functional Speech Disorder"—has been constructed from the following papers: "Psychoanalytic Concepts of the Stutterer" (1943), "A Social-Psychiatric Therapy for the Stutterer" (1944), "The Mother in the Etiology of the Stutterer" (1951), "The Nature and Treatment of Stuttering" (1950), "The Psychoanalysis of Stuttering" (1958), "Notes on the Early Stages in the Development of Stuttering" (1959), and "Further Contributions to the Concept of Stuttering" (1962).

Part II includes papers on a variety of related themes. A number of the clinical cases that gave rise to these studies were patients with speech disorders: Chapter 8, "Observations on a Primary Form of Anhedonia" (1949); Chapter 9, "A Deterrent in the Study and Practice of Medicine" (1953); Chapter 10, "The Rebirth Motif in Homosexuality and Its Teleological Significance" (1956); Chapter 11, "On the Meaning of Agoraphilia" (1955); Chapter 12, "Federn's Annotation of Freud's Theory of Anxiety" (1963); and Chapter 13, "Dysautomatization: A Disorder of Preconscious Ego Functioning" (1968).

This book should be of interest to mental health professionals, especially psychoanalysts, clinical psychologists, clinical social workers, speech therapists, counselors and guidance teachers.

Comments by some of the discussants at this meeting are presented in the following section.

In the ensuing ten years, Dr. Glauber spent about half of his time in research and treatment of stuttering, focusing on the problem of specificity. Up to 1956 he regularly found several very common factors, the body-phallus identity in which the mouth is the mediatus—the urinary excretory, which he thought was very significant; also the genetic factors; the family constellation, since it is organized almost entirely on the basis of symbiosis and it is not only the child participating in the symbiosis but also the marital partners. This is one chain of symbiotic relationship which very often is proved by an analysis of a significant member of the family—the mother. In Dr. Glauber's research on this problem of specificity, he has looked through many case histories of mothers in allied groups of alcoholics, schizophrenics, and perverts to see in what way the mother of the stutterer resembled or differed from these related groups. His strong impression was that the mothers and their rejection, whatever the basis, was consistent in these allied groups. The degrees of ambivalence found in the mother and the stutterer is a primary factor.

In January of 1966, Dr. Glauber wrote to a colleague in relation to treatment and cure, "Here I only can say that drive-defense psychology cannot comprehend a disorder involving an ego automatism, even though it serves as a fixation point for a later character disorder; but a more sophisticated ego psychology can. Neither is classical analytic therapy suitable for the needed cure. I am in the process of devising a parameter for analysis and/or else— a para-analytic speech therapy, both based on analytic insight into the essential difficulty plus a better understanding of the rationale of successful non-analytic therapy."

In Dr. Glauber's last paper, "Dysautomatization: A Disorder of Preconscious Ego Functioning" (1968), he spells out his final thinking on specificity. "I will recapitulate my view that stuttering, per se, is a two-fold disorder. It is first a symptom in the sense of a fixation or a traumatic disturbance of the rhythm of a psychosomatic automatism, as well as a fixation of the defense which also contributes to the rhythm disturbance, both during the advanced learning phase of the function. Secondarily, later conflicts of the

Preface

The selection of papers in this book, published between 1943 and 1968, represents I. Peter Glauber's special interests: psychoanalytic research, treatment, and the theory of preconscious ego functioning and ego defects. Focusing on the symptom of stuttering, he developed a profound understanding of character disorders and of the pregenital and narcissistic aspects of the neuroses.

Dr. Glauber's understanding of the symptom of stuttering as having its roots in the preoedipal phase of development, as well as his emphasis on ego defects and developmental arrests, anticipated many of the current trends in psychoanalysis. His treatment approach, with its stress on the psychiatric team and on psychoanalytically oriented psychotherapy, also anticipated current psychotherapeutic trends.

Dr. Glauber presented his paper, "The Mother in the Etiology of Stuttering," at a meeting of the New York Psychoanalytic Society. He stated: "In presenting this paper tonight on the memorial occasion of Dr. Federn's death, while altogether coincidental, I think it requires a word from me by way of gratitude to the memory of Dr. Federn, because he was very helpful to me with this particular paper. I was impressed, above all, by his great capacity for identification with a writer as well as with the reader. And I recall the fact that in one of his papers, he mentioned that one cannot understand anything unless one has the capacity to identify. To him it was not only a cliche. To him it was something that he lived. And I think, at a time when our world is suffering from so much splintering, as well as our analytic world, it is well to remember that Federn gave us a remedy—the ability to distinguish between sick and healthy narcissism, and the ability, particularly, to identify. So my first gratitude is to the memory of Dr. Paul Federn."

ing questions, as well as regrets that Dr. Glauber's professional life was so short.

W. Clifford M. Scott, M.D.
Montreal, Quebec, Canada

complex subject; and lucidity of presentation. Among the intensely practical issues are the role of psychoanalysis as such in treatment, the concept of a "family neurosis," and the usefulness of a "team approach." (Needless to say, the essays in the second part ranging from subjects such as "Anhedonia" to "Federn's Annotation of Freud's Theory of Anxiety" are substantial psychoanalytic contributions, whether or not immediately related to the main theme.)

Few (if any!) psychoanalysts of high attainment have had the depth and breadth of experience with speech disorders which Dr. Glauber had. It is therefore, a rare opportunity to read the crystallization of this experience in this book, following many years of thoughtful and deeply informed consideration.

Leo Stone, M.D.
New York, NY

Foreword

W. Clifford M. Scott, M.D.—   Leo Stone, M.D.—

Peter Glauber's untimely death in 1966 robbed psychoanalysis of one of those diligent workers on the "psychotic core" in neuroses and character disorders. His work with speech defects, and with disorders of learning and of thinking, lead him to write a series of condensed papers, very worth reading and pondering upon in the form edited by his wife. In the background of his work was the latent dialogue between Freud and Federn whose views were based on quite different types of clinical experience. This dialogue concerning the relation of the development of anxiety and the ego is outlined in one chapter, but the implications of this dialogue in clinical practice are evident in each of the other twelve chapters.

Dr. Glauber's condensed style leads to rereading. Each rereading leads to a stimulating productive dialogue with the author. Too few psychoanalysts have written an autobiography outlining the development of their professional career. This book can be read with great profit as Dr. Glauber's professional autobiography. The reader will be left with much information and with provok-

(continued next page)

I have recently had the privilege of perusing this impressive book-length collection of the late Dr. Glauber's psychoanalytic essays on the problems of speech, focussed on the wide-spread phenomenon of stuttering. The first half of the book consists of selected papers, explicitly devoted to various theoretical and clinical aspects of this important subject. The second part includes a wider range of psychoanalytic subjects. Nevertheless, at times by direct clinical reference in their texts, or by the depth—psychological considerations with which they deal, their organic and enriching connectedness with the main theme is strikingly maintained. Indeed, in the final paper ("Dysautomatization: A Disorder of Preconscious Ego Functioning), stuttering is conceptualized as the prototype of this phenomenon.

Since I knew Peter Glauber as a fellow analytic student in the days of candidacy, and then as a respected colleague and personal friend, I would have expected this book to exhibit the qualities which are conspicuously present: thorough scholarship; balanced and sane evaluations of the many different elements intrinsic in a

(continued next page)

Grateful acknowledgment is made to the publishers and editors of the journals and books in which the material in this volume first appeared. To:

- Family Service Association of America for "The Nature and Treatment of Stuttering."
- Harper and Row for "The Psychoanalysis of Stuttering" in *Stuttering: A Symposium.*
- *International Journal of Psycho-Analysis* for "The Rebirth Motif in Homosexuality," and "Dysautomatization: A Disorder of Preconscious Ego Functioning."
- International Universities Press for "Projective Tests in a Private Service for the Treatment of Functional Speech Disorder"; "Freud's Contribution on Stuttering: Their Relation to Some Current Insights"; "On the Meaning of Agoraphilia"; "Federn's Annotation of Freud's Theory of Anxiety"; "Notes on the Early Stages in the Development of Stuttering"; and "Further Contributions to the Concept of Stuttering."
- *Journal of the American Psychoanalytic Association* for "Freud's Contributions on Stuttering: Their Relation to Some Current Insights"; "On the Meaning of Agoraphilia"; and "Federn's Annotation of Freud's Theory of Anxiety."
- National Association of Social Workers for "A Social Psychiatric Therapy for the Stutterer."
- *Psychoanalytic Quarterly* for "Observations of a Primary Form of Anhedonia" and "A Deterrent in the Study and Practice of Medicine."

Acknowledgments

My deep feelings of gratitude go to several of my friends and colleagues who patiently supported me in my desire to put together Dr. Glauber's papers in book form as a memorial to his unflagging devotion to the theory and practice of psychoanalysis with special emphasis on the research and treatment of the stuttering syndrome.

Dr. Edward Holtzman and Dr. Peter Brundl helped me in a practical way by sorting out with me the most important papers of thirty years of accumulation of material—a good deal of which had found its way into his published papers.

My warm thanks to M. Masud R. Kahn of London who made arrangements for the publication of "Dysautomatization"; to Dr. H. Robert Blank for his help in writing a brief summary of it and to Dr. Peter Laderman who read the paper at a meeting of the Westchester Psychoanalytic Society.

For the sympathetic and editing assistance by my very dear friend and colleague, Mrs. Sylvia Grobe, I am especially grateful.

My everlasting gratitude to Oscar Nemon, sculptor, of London, whose bust of Dr. Glauber is a joy to me and my family. My thanks to Peter Grobe for his splendid photography of this bust.

My deep appreciation of the secretarial work of Mrs. Sadie Cullo, beyond the call of duty.

My grateful appreciation to the Mental Health Materials Center especially to Mr. Alex Sareyan and to Mae Kanazawa, editor, for their patience and interest.

Thanks are also due to Katharine B. Wolpe, librarian, Abraham A. Brill Library, New York Psychoanalytic Institute, for her assistance in locating references and for the excellent index which she has prepared for this material.

Contents

Part I
A Psychoanalytic Understanding of Stuttering

Part II
Other Selected Papers

Published by Human Sciences Press Inc., 72 Fifth Avenue, New York, NY 10011.
No part of this book may be reproduced in any form by any means without the permission of the author.

Printed in the United States of America.
23456789 987654321

Library of Congress Cataloging in Publication Data

Glauber, I. Peter
  Stuttering A psychoanalytic understanding.
  Bibliography: p.
  Includes index.
    1. Stuttering—Psychological aspects—Collected
works. 2. Psychoanalysis—Collected works.
I. Glauber, Helen M. II. Title. [DNLM:
1. Neurotic disorders—Collected works. 2. Stutter-
ing—Collected Works. 3. Psychoanalytic
theory—Collected works. WM 475 G551p]
RC424,G58 1982   616.85'54   82-8125
ISBN 0-89885-154-8   AACR2

STUTTERING
A Psychoanalytic Understanding

I. Peter Glauber, M.D.

Edited by
Helen M. Glauber

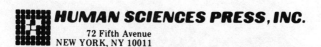 **HUMAN SCIENCES PRESS, INC.**
72 Fifth Avenue
NEW YORK, NY 10011

the interest and attention of more heterogeneous sources of investigators than has any other human dysfunction.... We are particularly grateful to Dr. Glauber for his calling to our attention Freud's early study of this ailment in his patient Frau Emmy Von N, a study which, as Dr. Glauber points out, is rich in observations and historical interest."

Dr. Henry I. Schneer: "This year of the Freud centennial, it would be hard to find a more appropriate person to discuss the subject of stuttering than Dr. Glauber. Among psychoanalysts today, he is one who has consistently and persistently explored the psychodynamic foundations of stuttering, and has given us more and more reason to show that stuttering is primarily causatively a disturbance of the mental apparatus and not the vocal apparatus, although there are still many who direct therapy to the vocal apparatus.

Coriat was said to have taken the analysis of stuttering further than Freud, and I believe Glauber has taken it still further, and has also contributed to another area of psychoanalysis, ego psychology. The line of psychoanalytic investigation in Dr. Glauber's paper is demonstrated from the first hint of Freud that stuttering may be a displacement upwards of conflicts over excremental conflicts. In a reported discussion of Federn's paper on Asthma, regarding narcissism and oral development levels, to Fenichel's classification of stuttering as a pregenital conversion, to Coriat's representation of stuttering as an oral perversion, and finally to Glauber's refinement of the neurosis perversion problem set forth by elucidating the mother-child symbiosis, the passivity activity aspect of stuttering as an interference to the ego emergence along with the part-object identification and the body-breast phallus equation. I'm sure that the Glaubers, Dr. and Mrs., can adduce many clinical cases."

Dr. Ernst Kris: "The material presented by Dr. Glauber, and I would say many clinical expressions by others in relation to tics or others what Freud calls fixation neurosis in his comment of 1913, what we used to call a pregenital conversion neurosis, indicates that we have here ego structures which seem to be characterized by two features, probably more. One is, I believe, a very early onset to dominance. That is to say, that same prematurity which we find in the whole range of anything which approaches the obsessive compulsive disorders, so a very premature attempt at control, and a very early and radical breakdown of these premature attempts. Hence, we would find then that essential ego functions like speech, facial expression or in the obsessional compulsive neurosis itself, thought processes are not only subject to regressive expressions, but are sexualized or instinctualized to an unusual extent, as if the essential ego functions, namely to keep certain functions free from sexualization, would have miscarried, and it is in line with Dr. Glauber's ideas, and I think I could concur from my own experiences in somewhat different fields, that the disturbances of this nature must have some relation to disturbances of object relations, which then must be combined with specific experiences in relation to oral aggression, and then with that I would call a different pace of development of the organization of sexuality and aggression in the small child."

Dr. Bertram D. Lewin, wrote in a personal letter October 11, 1956, to Dr. Glauber, "It was a bit late in the evening when I settled down to read your paper, but that can't be the only reason I found myself letting myself go and enjoying it. I was surprised to learn so much about Frau Emmy. It certainly is there for one who can read it. . . . I certainly am impressed by what you have been able to bring together concerning the topic. Maybe you could collect your papers on stuttering or rewrite them into a more available book form?"

Some comments by colleagues on "Dysautomatization":

Dr. H. Robert Blank wrote, "You will be interested to know that my second group of residents and fellows in child psychiatry have already read the paper and have found it most instructive, especially because we have been discussing quite a few young psychotic children in our in-patient service who have prominent speech disturbances. What pertinent points Peter made in his discussion of trauma!"

Dr. Leopold Bellak, of Postdoctoral Program for Study and Research in Psychology of New York University wrote, "Our whole research project revolves around the study of ego functions, and the idea of automaticity and its disturbance is a very important one for us. . . . I found a number of formulations in Peter's paper particularly useful, such as the facultative functions."

On March 29, 1961, Dr. M. Masud R. Khan, in a personal communication, had this to say: "your paper on anhedonia is very close to the problems I am dealing with. In fact, it is, as it were, the other side of the penny. The extreme psychic masochism that one clinically meets with in the 'transference emotionality' of the schizoid patient is a screen-affect against a more distressing symptom, namely, incapacity for pleasurable affects. One of the very difficult clinical tasks, in my experience, with these patients is how to wean them from this addiction to psychic masochism—which is used both narcissistically and . . . heavily eroticised—and enable them to tolerate real anxiety and aggression, which is a precondition for enjoyment of pleasurable affects in a healthy ego. I think the answer to this problem most probably will derive, as you suggest, from a closer study of ego-boundary phenomena and their developmental vicissitudes. The craving for pleasure in these patients is also a relevant issue. Recently I was intrigued to find this problem in a drug addict who had a mild stammer as well."

Subsequently, on October 5, 1961, he again wrote to remark about Dr. Glauber's article on stuttering: "May I say how very cogently you have stated the psycho-pathology of the stutterer, as well as clearly reviewed the significant literature on the subject. What has particularly interested me are your own contributions towards the theme. I find your shift of emphasis in the etiology of the stutterer to early ego defect and arrest both clinically valid and theoretically useful.

"As you can well imagine, I find many correspondences between the personality schema which you have established for the stutterer and the one I have been trying to define in terms of the schizoid character. To me both the correspondences and differences are equally significant. And I am very impressed by the way you have related regression in ego level to the phenomenology of the stuttering syndrome. When I was reading your paper I was very much reminded of Dr. Greenacre's paper in the International Journal where she discusses the interaction between certain physical traits of pre-genital patterning with early formation of the ego defense mechanisms. I am sure you are familiar with this paper. . . ."

Part I

A Psychoanalytic Understanding of Stuttering

Chapter 1

Stuttering, Speech, and the Ego

Stuttering is a symptom of an ego dysfunction. A symptom is an unsuccessful attempt to resolve an unconscious conflict. The conflict reflected in stuttering is between a wish to speak and a fear of speaking or a wish to be mute. Because both contributors to the conflict find expression in the symptom, mental tension is reduced, but the conflict is not resolved, and the stuttering is an indicator of that.

A genuine resolution of the conflict would lead either to smooth speech or uncontested silence. When we listen to the stutterer we note both aspects. In various stutterers, or in one stutterer at various times, one or the other wish may predominate. Accordingly, the empathic listener will note that at times he knows easily what the stutterer is saying; at other times, when the stutterer's dominant wish is not to communicate, the effect on the listener is almost as if the stutterer had not spoken at all, as if he had been completely mute.

The stutter—a bit of character in action—is a trait in its earliest forms. It is attached to a physiological automatism, speech, serving the function of expression and communication. In origin, it is a preverbal gesture which is a condensation of the total ego. Hence, it is often the only complaint. I agree with Fenichel (1945) that stuttering occurs in a condition called a pregenital conversion neurosis. The pregenital refers to the developmental stage during which the conflict that produced the symptom originates. Conversion refers to the fact that a psychic conflict is transformed into physical expression via the functioning of a physical organ. We call the condition a neurosis because the stutterer unconsciously accepts his/her symptom as one of the terms of an attempted settlement between contending components of the personality. Apparently an inner threat is felt as a greater evil, and the conscious suffering, or symptoms, as a lesser evil.

In my view, the most significant predisposing factor in stuttering is serious trauma during the early months of life. By trauma I mean not an isolated experience but an unhealthy environment from which flow disturbing stimuli varying from the subliminal to those that may threaten life. Broadly speaking, the trauma consists of inadequate mothering during the most helpless period in the child's life.

The symbiotic tie with the mother is crucial in the genesis of the disorder and a prototype for difficulties in interpersonal relations. The factor of separation anxiety in this primary identification cannot be overemphasized. I have been struck by the strength of the tie to a mother who is anxious and ambivalent, who weans even while she nurses. My studies of the mother-child relationship led me to the analysis of the mother, the father, and the total family constellation. Indeed, I have been led to characterize stuttering as essentially a family disorder.

Stuttering is the principal symptom, then, in a neurosis that involves speech. Now, speech has no organ of its own; it uses many borrowed organs, organs having totally different functions. This basic fact suggests a connection between the primary functions of these organs and the added functions. These organs comprise not only the mouth and throat but also the rest of the gastrointestinal tract, as well as the entire respiratory system, including the diaphragm. The functions of these organ systems are self-evident. In addition, we must include the general body musculature, for in observing a stutterer we see not only tonic and clonic spasms in the mouth and throat muscles that destroy the smooth functioning of speech, but also similar spasms of the face, neck, and general body musculature.

A number of observations about speech and its development are relevant for the understanding of stuttering. The well-known transitions from babbling, lalling, echolalia to communicative speech represent steps in a change of direction from narcissistic to object-related expression, a change that marks the emergence of the ego as a separate mental structure. Speech thus becomes an ego function along with perception, thinking, and reality testing.

Before the acquisition of speech, the child is able to recognize and to love objects and to fear reality. Toward the end of the second year of life there are definite signs of a differentiation within the psychic apparatus—the emergence of the ego. Among a number of evidential factors such as improved locomotion and attempts at sphincter control, speech is the most significant. It is significant not only as a sign of ego emergence, but also, as an instrument for its further maturation. Included in this process are advances in the development of reality testing. Words permit more exact communication with others and more precise anticipation by trial actions. Such anticipations evolve into thinking and help consolidate consciousness. Thinking is an advance over the earlier so-called consciousness without words, which is recognizable in later regressive states as "preconscious fantasy thinking." These early or pre-ego states play an important role in the psychopathology of stuttering. The "thinking" before ego development is primary-process thinking familiar to us because it characterizes our dreams. It ignores all the rules of logic, equates parts with wholes, and sees similarities as identities.

Speech evolving as the symbol for things gradually helps to develop the capacity for understanding and rationality in the handling of external reality and the instinctual drives. Speech also helps to control anxiety by causing a shift from emotional fantasy to sober reality.

The acquisition of the ability to speak is experienced as a powerful achievement. The child endows words and thoughts with a magical omnipotence having the power to charm people and even fate itself to do his bidding. Words and thoughts become magical gestures for the attainment of a multiplicity of needs, hostile and libidinal, as well as destructive reactions to frustration. It is these archaic aspects of thinking and of speech as reflections of the primitive or pre-ego states that constitute essential elements in the psychopathology of the personality and speech of the stutterer.

Our earliest thinking is in accord with the pleasure principle; it is dominated by the wish to have pleasure and avoid pain, and is unlike the later logical, organized, and more adjusted thinking which comes with the advent of the ego and the faculty of speech.

The fact is that, even after speech and logical thinking and the reality principle have been established, prelogical thinking still remains operative. Normally repressed, we see it return in states of ego regression and in other conditions. This kind of thinking does not serve to help prepare for future actions but becomes, instead, a substitute for unpleasant reality.

Thus the faculty of speech is burdened by the possibility of having to express primitive, magical id impulses and associated emotions as well as primitive ego states of perception and execution. The expression in thoughts and words of superego precursors burdens the ego even further.

Our starting point in understanding the psychopathology of stuttering is in understanding that all the components of the unconscious mind—id, ego, and superego—may be represented through the urge to speak. Speech represents a concrete action, a product of the drives before they were tamed into the ego function of communication. Accordingly, speech is the self in action: the self exposed in acting out a libidinal or aggressive drive. Speech may thus represent the id or the primitive ego in the service of the id. It may express an attack, or a wish to be attacked, in an oral, anal, phallic manner; to exhibit one's self or to be a voyeur; to wish to hurt or to get masochistic pleasure; to be loved or to be reprimanded. It may also represent the primitive superego which derives a large part of its energy from the id.

We know from folklore that to name a thing is to master it. From the psychology of dreams (Freud, 1900) we have learned that to speak signifies to be alive and to love, and to be mute means to be dead or to hate. Tausk (1933) suggested that one reason the paranoid patient believes others can read his thoughts is that his words were first given to him by his parents and that somehow words are still not quite his own possession. This relates to another archaic notion that what happens to oneself causes the same thing to happen to the object. In this way speech may become a "magical gesture": by saying something to another person the latter may be found to do the same thing, or the same thing may affect him as the speaker.

A very important meaning of speech stems from a later, anal, period of development. Here, words are equatable with dangerous anal products which may kill the object. They must be held back or, like any dangerous tool, handled very cautiously. In this context belong obscene words and oaths, which may represent an anal assault or a violently sexual, i.e., sadistic, attack. When conflicts over such acts or fantasies are projected upon the articulatory apparatus, stuttering may result. The symptom here, as elsewhere, then represents partly the breakthrough of a forbidden expression and partly the attempt to abort it.

Although the trauma that predisposes someone to stutter occurs during the preoedipal phase, problems of later developmental periods are also invariably involved because an inability to solve them frequently leads to their regressive reorganization under the primacy of earlier levels of libido and ego functioning. In stuttering, the regression may be to any one of the earlier phases. For example, a boy having many fears and conflicts about his masturbation gave up the practice and took up an earlier pleasurable preoccupation with anal activities. It was only when these were blocked that he regressed to the oral level and developed a stutter. His stutter represented phallic and anal elements distorted by the dominant oral expression.

At the phallic stage, speech is directly involved in the oedipal conflict. Here, to speak, or to speak well, means to be potent; to be unable to speak, to be castrated. To the boy it means phallic competition with his father. In that type of situation the tongue becomes the symbol for the phallus. The castration complex is here represented by the many legends, based on unconscious fantasies, of punishment by means of the tongue being cut out.

Another significant unconscious meaning of speech is that it serves the exhibitionistic impulse. This is related to ambition (Lewin, 1933), which has also another root to be mentioned presently. The urge to exhibit may be countered by a reaction formation resulting in an inhibition of speech. This inhibition is similar to the fear of blushing, stage fright, and fears in social situations in general. Back of the urge to exhibit is a desire for the magical influencing of the audience through the omnipotence of thoughts and words. This is not unrelated to the perverse sexual pleasure of exhibitionism. The need to exhibit oneself has a multiplicity of aims. For one thing, there is the ever-present desire for reassurance against the ubiquitous castration fears; for another, equally potent and related, the narcissistic need to be loved. Acquiring these reassurances in an environment felt to be hostile is a complicated effort fraught with doubts and dangers. Common unconscious reactions may be stated in the following terms: "I wish to influence this audience or charm them, be applauded, or else kill them. My power over them may be overwhelming. I fear it myself, or else they may fear it and retaliate. I must stop before I kill them. Or I must stop before they see through me" (Fenichel, 1945). Obviously, there are here strong motivations for proceeding with speech as well as for attempting to halt it.

The most significant zone for speech and its disorders is the oral zone. It represents a very early period of libido and ego functioning, preceding that of speech. Molded by the processes of nursing and weaning, the oral zone retains a large part of their influence during the period of speech development. This zone stands in close relation to the very earliest stirrings of the ego when it was still conceived predominantly in magical terms. The major pleasure experience here is in terms of sucking and chewing; relationships with the outside world are in terms of swallowing if the objects are "good" and spitting them out if they are "bad." There is an associated and subsidiary reflex tendency to evacuate immediately or shortly after ingestion; this also leaves lingering psychological traces. Between the world felt as so many variants of food and the final recognition of objects as human individuals, the developing child experiences his environment through a number of transitional animate and inanimate objects. This period is rich in what are known as fixation points—early instinctual and ego patterns from which the individual cannot free himself to evolve further and to which he regresses when later developmental problems prove to be too intractable. When that happens, the later forms of ego and instinctual expressions fall under the primacy or dominance of the earlier fixated patterns and become distorted thereby.

The oral zone, so important in the biological economy, necessarily carries a very large pleasure premium throughout life, but especially so in the first few years. At the very beginning, oral pleasure flows from the oral and respiratory functions as the two merge in nursing. To this is soon added the satisfactions from the aural or auditory zones—the sound of mother's voice and the baby's own undifferentiated noises. The nature of these pleasures are incorporative as well as autoerotic. Incorporative wishes may have a libidinal or a hostile aim. The latter would then be equatable with killing the object. Using the articulatory apparatus may then signify that words are introjected objects, that killing the object and the words are one and the same. One result may be a speech inhibition.

Oral erogeneity, accentuated for various reasons, may lead to ambition in the field of speech. The expression of the ambition may be quite variable. In a direct way it may lead to a deep interest in languages, philology, or linguistics. A deep interest in speech may also follow in a compensatory way upon a transient speech disorder long forgotten.

Speech in the service of ambition may acquire an exaggerated importance from sources other than pure oral erogeneity. It may represent competitiveness based on the need for self-aggrandizement or narcissistic enhancement: to make more noise than the other fellow, to stand up and be counted, to show that one has a voice in all matters, etc.

A seemingly curious but quite significant need to speak much may depend upon a need to eat excessively. This in turn often represents an identification with one who wishes to eat aggressively, i.e., it is a defense against a wish to be eaten. The latter is not an uncommon and very serious regressive reaction against a host of fearsome tasks and attainments requiring a courageous, active role. Another need to eat and talk in excess is more simple: to feel on an equal footing with adults. Still another aspect of oral ambition is the imbibing of words by hearing and reading. In the last instance the need to speak may also be inhibited more directly; but in all instances the inhibitions are reactive to excesses which are felt to be dangerous.

A few remarks on the unconscious connection between speech and breathing are in order. Physiologically, nursing enhances the respiratory function. Another connection is that breathing and smelling, which are equivalent in the unconscious, also express the idea of incorporation. This respiratory erotism parallels the oral, possibly explaining the close resemblance between asthma and stuttering. Exerting power through control of the breath is a frequent component of cults of magic. On the other hand, the expression "breath of life" is an indication of the identity of the two. The fact of smothering is expressed in the birth process and in suckling, and thereafter remains connected unconsciously with every experience of danger and its affect, anxiety. A frequent experience of the stuttering child while speaking is a sudden spasm of the diaphragm as it is gradually relaxing during exhalation. He suddenly inhales, thus interrupting his speech, which is possible only during exhalation.

Chapter 2

A Review of the Literature

A review of the psychoanalytic literature on stuttering must begin with Freud, not alone out of deference to the discoverer and founder of psychoanalysis but because his contributions in this field—a fact generally unrecognized—touch on the major aspects of the syndrome. They consist of a lengthy case presentation,* several pithy theoretical statements—all to be found in his writings— and an oral statement reported to me in a personal communication.

Freud, so far as I know, made only two statements on the subject. In 1901 he distinguished between slips of the tongue and stuttering caused by embarrassment, saying that the latter "speech disturbances cannot any longer be described as slips of the tongue because what they effect is not the individual word, but the rhythm and execution of the whole speech.... But here too... it is a question of an internal conflict which is betrayed to us by the disturbance in speech" (pp. 100–101). Needless to say, this is an important distinction, for it points to the constricted character of a slip of the tongue as contrasted with the more global nature of stuttering. The distinction is worth emphasizing: I have noticed that sometimes the same therapeutic approach is vainly applied to the stutter as to the parapraxis.

Freud's second remark is contained in a letter he wrote to Ferenczi in 1915 (see Jones, 1955, p. 183), wherein he mentioned that "stammering could be caused by a displacement to speech of conflicts over excremental functions." This idea represented then,

---

*A detailed discussion of Freud's contributions to stuttering as revealed through his description of the case of Frau Emmy von N. (Breuer and Freud, 1893–1895) will be found in Chapter 3—Ed.

and probably still does, a basic foundation stone in the psycho-analytic orientation on stuttering. Fenichel (1945) elaborated on it as follows:

> Psychoanalysis of stutterers reveals the anal-sadistic universe of wishes as the basis of the symptom . . . . Speaking means, first, the utterance of obscene, especially anal, words and, second, an aggressive act directed against the listener . . . . In dreams, to speak is the symbol of life, and to be mute the symbol of death (Freud, 1900). The same symbolism holds true in stuttering . . . . "Words can kill," and stutterers are persons who unconsciously think it necessary to use so dangerous a weapon with care (p. 312).

Fenichel also included three other component impulses that played a part in stuttering: the phallic, oral, and exhibitionistic.

On the basis of what Freud stated, we can understand the generally held concept that, while the symptomatology of the stutterer is in the nature of a conversion, the patient's mental structure corresponds to that of a compulsive neurotic (Fenichel, 1945). However, looked at more closely, each of the components of the concept requires modification. The conversion is not the hysterical one stemming from oedipal conflicts, but is pregenital in origin; and the compulsion neurosis is, as is not infrequent, a defense against the underlying orality as well as a regression from genitality. Thus both character and symptoms are cut out of the same cloth.

In 1923, A. A. Brill spoke before a group of speech teachers on the subject of speech disturbances in nervous and mental diseases. His paper, in nontechnical language, touched on so many aspects of stuttering so succinctly that it may well serve as a bird's-eye view of the psychoanalytic orientation on stuttering at the time. Brill began with the problems of treatment and stated that experience had gradually made him less enthusiastic though not pessimistic regarding it. At a large clinic he had interviewed over 600 patients. He had treated 69 from a few months to a year and over; the ages ranged from 15 to 51. It is not explicitly stated, but we can assume that the classical psychoanalytic treatment was not used in the clinic, though psychoanalytic understanding was utilized. Most of the patients he regarded as much improved or cured when they left. He followed them up through their yearly communications.

Elaborating on the prognosis of the stuttering after treatment, Brill emphasized the tendency to recurrence. After 11 years, he found only 5 of the 69 patients doing entirely well. One of the 5 regressed in his speech following being drafted into the Army. Brill added that he could be very busy if he took care of all the stutterers "cured" by others. He found the prognosis among young children much better. These could usually be cured if treated properly. "Like every other psychoneurotic symptom, speech disturbances can be cured quicker and more thoroughly when they have not become interwoven in the whole being of the person" (p. 132). Another group having a favorable treatment outlook are psychoneurotics who began stuttering at a later age; still another consists of psychopaths and mild mental defectives in whom transient speech disturbances were observed.

One question on which psychoanalysts appear to be divided is the need for supplementary speech training. Brill belonged to the group who believe in training and gave the usual rationale of that group, namely, that the patients have acquired bad "habits" of speech which need to be "untrained" or "retrained."

Brill made some interesting comments regarding the sex ratio of distribution—the well-known fact that there are at least four or five males to one female stutterer—adding that this was in contrast to the ratio in psychoneurosis in general. I do not believe that he meant that the two groups are in inverse ratio, but rather that more females than males have the classical neuroses. I do not know the current statistics about the latter, but my impression is that the difference, if any, is not marked.

Regarding the basis for the sexual distribution, Brill quoted Jespersen's (1922) theory, which he apparently accepted, that the male tends to go to extremes regarding his speech. He is normally less fluent and shows greater preponderance in speech disturbances. The female has more control of her speech but a smaller vocabulary. The male tends to be more quiet and silent but more aggressive in his thoughts. The female talks about simpler things, encounters less criticism. Present-day competitive civilization leaves little time for speech to the male. The female, on the other hand, according to Jespersen, has no need for involved thinking, as she is in constant close relationship with the simple human being, the child. She can cook, bake, crochet, and talk at the same time. The preponderance of speech disturbance as a psychoneurotic symptom in the male is thus only an exaggeration of his normal activity. The female's speech is more fluent and not as vulnerable as the male's. In my view, this concept may be characterized as more anthropologic than psychoanalytic.

In common with all psychoanalysts, Brill did not consider stuttering a symptom of a classical neurosis; he was struck by the features of introversion, some paranoid tincturing of the personality, and autoerotic and narcissistic fixations.

Before concluding, he mentioned two or three other significant and practical points: Speech disturbances disappear when the individual feels free to express himself fully, that is, when he can give and take emotions in a normal way. This is a way of saying that in order to be cured the stutterer must accomplish mastery over his characteristic tendency to turn upon himself—to introvert his affects and keep them dissociated from the realm of the intellect. The dissociation is a major defense and overcoming it a crucial step in the analysis.

Brill mentioned the fundamental fact of neurosis, that the symptom unconsciously represents a morbid gain for the patient who then refuses to give it up, also unconsciously; and that the stutterer, like other chronic neurotics, utilizes his stuttering to escape from various difficulties and stutters more when confronted with disagreeable tasks, the phenomenon of secondary gain.

Brill regarded prophylaxis as more important than treatment. Because many children begin to show signs of stuttering at an early age, study of the behavior of the parents toward the child is indicated. He advocated bringing the child in closer contact with other children, suggesting a parental tie that is unhealthy because it is too close. He cautioned against impressing the child that it has a malady, thus causing self-consciousness. He was impressed by a hereditary predisposition and by the fact that stuttering is one of the most intractable of symptoms, especially in the adult stutterer.

Brill's statements on therapy and prophylaxis as related here are essentially true in the light of current insights, at least in my experience. However, they are oversimplified, partly owing to the requirements of his paper and partly because they antedate the insights acquired in the intervening years.

Among psychoanalysts, perhaps no one has written more about stuttering than Isadore H. Coriat, beginning in 1915 and continuing for almost 30 years. The most important of his writings was his monograph, *Stammering: A Psychoanalytic Interpretation*, which appeared in 1928. His writings, though reflecting in the main the psychoanalytic insights of his time, also included important ideas and emphases of his own. His contribution consisted mainly in placing in the forefront the dynamic factor of oral libido, an emphasis that was altogether new. He marshaled findings from various sources. He compared the reflex experiments on the newborn infant's tendencies to suck, bite, and incorporate with the oral activities in adult stutterers. These findings paralleled reconstructions of infantile states in the pregenital neuroses. He studied observations on the mouth activities of older nurslings who sucked after they were fed. He also compared oral libidinal Pavlovian conditioned reflexes with the idea of the illusory nipple among stutterers. He studied his patients' associations, his clinical observations of them, and their clear, often literal, dreams and fantasies. He concluded that the basic causative factor in stuttering is accentuated libido within the mouth. In my opinion, that contribution stands today as valid, even though Coriat's total evaluation and interpretation of that fact may be questioned as insufficiently inclusive, and despite his tendency to undervalue other factors. For him, the role of oral aggression was a minor one; and he hardly considered the roles of the ego and of narcissism beyond mentioning them.

To Coriat, stuttering consists essentially of a persistence into adult life of infantile nursing activities. He often reiterated that careful observation would prove that the stutterer's attempts to speak reveal motor patterns of an act of nursing at an illusory nipple. He described cannibalistic muscular patterns, anal-retentive and anal-expulsive patterns, and placed them in a secondary role. He was able to trace certain character traits of the stutterer from the oral fixations, underscoring the fact that in many instances these traits were almost as infantile as the erotism from which they emerged. In the rhythmic character of nursing he saw the root of the fluctuations in the speech and the labile emotional swings in the personality as a whole. Similarly, the obstinacy and verbal "constipation" were traceable to anal erotism.

His great emphasis on the dominant role of the pleasure principle in the symptom in terms of the excessive concentration of libido in the mouth led him to picture stuttering fundamentally as a perversion. This fact was evidenced also in his use of phrases found in Abraham (1916)—mouth pollutions and oral masturbation. Coriat stated that stuttering is not a genuine conversion in a pregenital neurosis, but a neurosis in which the original pregenital tendencies have persisted from an early organization of the libido. Consequently, the beginnings of stuttering in early childhood are not of a psychoneurotic nature; it is only through the persistence of early oral and anal activities that stuttering becomes a neurotic symptom. This distinction may be analogous to the nonanalytic, descriptive approach which speaks of "primary" and "secondary" stuttering. There is no question that the personality of the stutterer when fully developed fulfills the requirements of a neurosis. Coriat must have been quite aware of that because he wrote (1928, p. 5) that the motivating mechanism producing the stutter is unconscious and the only conscious reaction was anxiety and fear. In a genuine perversion those affects are not present or prominent. It is obvious that Coriat saw perverse *and* neurotic phenomena in the stutter and that he thought of these categories as not sharply distinguishable. He was aware of the double aspect of symptoms, including partial attempts at instinctual gratification and prohibition.

He believed that the defect resulted both from a resistance barrier between thoughts and vocal expression and from a compulsive repetition of the original nursing activities, rather than from the content of the thoughts themselves. Coriat thus approximated Freud's distinction between a slip of the tongue and stuttering, and added that the content of the symptom is not related to a specific thought content but to the special impulses which the unconscious equates with thoughts and words in general—notably nursing and biting wishes.

Coriat (1933) underscored the special significance of the castration complex in the female stutterer. "The tongue has become a displaced phallus. The inner conflict within the libidinal economy has become concentrated on the lingual organ for the purpose of unconsciously satisfying a masculine aim. The conflict is between wishes to have a phallus, to envy those that have it, to acquire it in a cannibalistic manner, and the reactions of disgust and guilt" (p. 255). We know now that these conflicts arise in relation to early parental ties to and separations from the mother, which become intensified at the height of the oedipal rivalry. The mother is accused as the earliest one responsible for the "fact" of castration. Unhealthy resolutions of this complex may lead either to interminable hatred of the mother or mother surrogates or to homosexual attachments.

Coriat (1943) wrote clearly and emphatically about the psychoanalytic treatment of stuttering. He advocated the use of psychoanalysis, although he was thoroughly aware of the many difficulties resulting from resistances. He was opposed to speech training because it dealt with only one symptom and not with the total neurosis "and was thus inadequate and unscientific." Furthermore, he believed such training reinforced the oral erotism instead of relieving or lessening it. He advised directing the treatment against the resistances, which he recognized as "very severe because of the convergence of several factors. First is the narcissistic essence of the disorder; second, the reluctance to giving up the nursing pleasure in speech; third, the negativism or holding back acquired from the anal phase of development and expressed in oral terms. There is a parallelism between the difficulties encountered in analyzing the speech problem and the character traits due to the relative underdevelopment of the ego, at least as far as the oral and anal instinct gratification in early forms are concerned." He introduced a modification in the classical psychoanalytic technique, which he called "active therapy." In sum, this consisted of a marked reduction in the oral pleasures indulged in by these patients by ordering them to abstain from smoking, chewing gum, etc. This regimen, by helping to crystallize the resistance to the analytic treatment, aided in its resolution by demonstrating how these indulgences reinforced the oral difficulties of the stutterer.

Lewin in 1933 summarized his findings in two stutterers as follows: "In both patients the belief in the mother's phallus was unmistakable, as was their identification with it. It seemed that the oral-sadistic aim was the chief or central aim in their stammering, the ideational content—to ablate the breast—being displaced by way of the equation, breast-penis, to the phallus; that the fantasied incorporation of the phallus led to an identification of themselves with it; that this in turn led to the 'urethralization' and 'analization' of the mouth, the 'excrementalization' of the flow of speech, and to stammering . . . when the body becomes a phallus, the mouth becomes a urethra (and anus); and the stammering is a function of the reorganized libidinal arrangement" (p. 42). In recent years I have also been impressed by the importance of the visual and auditory spheres in speech pathology. Speaking situations frequently activate visual and auditory as well as oral conflicts which were first brought to the forefront in relation to primal-scene fantasies and experiences.

Somewhat later, Edward Glover (1939) said that stuttering "can be legitimately described as a 'mixed type' of psycho-neurosis . . . (arising) from disturbances at different psychic levels of function." Glover added that "It can appear as a functional reaction to mental stress either traumatic or as a result of emotional excitations, it can be induced by conflict without psycho-neurotic symptom formation. It can also be correlated with certain normal and psychotic manifestations" (p. 192).

Most of the findings have been on the metapsychological level of drives and their derivatives. In addition to the factors already mentioned, I have been impressed by a number of phenomena related to visual and auditory functions. These include primal-scene traumata of a visual or auditory nature leading to impulses to break the silence by sound or speech, impulses having strong oral-aggressive or aggressive-exhibitionistic quality or the opposite—inclinations to flee, to be mute. There are additional compulsions to speak and confess. It is possible to trace a connection between these early infantile traumata and later attempts to recollect these by means of acting out; i.e., phobic avoidance and counterphobic impulsion, especially in more dramatic speech situations involving an audience.

My own view, as it has developed in the last thirty years, has also favored the pregenital conversion idea. However, I formed a conviction from the very start, and it has grown with the years, that stuttering is primarily a disturbance affecting the ego. I base this conclusion on observations of older children, adolescents, and adults. In the younger children, the symptom first reflects anxiety during the act of speaking, which in turn develops into a more diffuse phobic anxiety for social or speech situations. It is more easily reversible then. Whether other ego manifestations are already present in the nascent state or are developed gradually only thereafter is not always easy to determine. But it is possible to recognize ego disturbances even in these small children. Two excerpts from the recent psychoanalytic literature exemplify thinking about stuttering similar to my own. The first is that of Wissa Wassef (1961), whose paper was summarized in *The Annual Survey of Psychoanalysis*, as follows:

> [Wassef] aims to show [in contrast to Fenichel] that to consider stammering in terms of a simple regression to the anal stage is to deal with only one variety of stammering, the obsessional type, to the exclusion of others in which anal material may not predominate or determine a psychological structure in which primitive elements have become integrated into a personality very different from that of the obsessional . . . .
>
> Furthermore, instinctual conflicts are on the oral and genital plane . . . . On another plane are archaic elements. The latter included sadistic conceptions of the primal scene and fusion of sadistic visual memories with thinking and speaking.
>
> The symptom of stammering condensed drives and defenses at all levels . . . . [It] represents both a fixation and a solution of the primitive conflict, [and] is also a progression in so far as there is an integration into the ego of conflicting ambivalent drives which still permit the realization of a triangular relationship . . . . It is as though the neurosis had achieved a solution on two levels which safeguarded the ego effectively . . . . [The analysis helped to attain a] transition from the partial to the total object relationship and integration of the primitive elements into the personality (pp. 158–160).

The second author is Charlotte Balkanyi (1961), who writes,

> During the analysis we became familiar with, and worked through, the structure of her stammer. Material thus obtained does not, however, fully reveal the cause of the symptom. This lay neither in the sensation of pleasure displaced from the anal and genital zones to the oral zone, nor in the predominance of exhibitionistic tendencies in the patient's whole sexuality. These I consider to be the motivation of

the condition, that is to say, its secondary functions . . . . Stammering is an independent pathological entity. *It is the dysfunction of the pre-conscious; the dysfunction of moulding affects into words* . . . . The psycho-analysis showed how the stammer, at first alien to her mental world, adapted itself to the service of various tendencies in the course of her development (p. 108).

The references to "two levels" in stuttering by Wassef and to an "independent pathological entity . . . and its secondary adaptation" by Balkanyi both suggest, as my own work does, fixation in archaic ego states more or less loosely synthesized with later more developed ego states. The fixation itself denotes an early defensive operation, and it is integrated in the service of current ego functioning. The recognizable anxieties are twofold: psychoneurotic-teleological-defensive, on the one hand; and, on the other, direct evidences of ego breakdown: depersonalization—"actual" existing anxieties.

One area of great interest with regard to stuttering is the field of physiology. Studies are being made of changes in the threshold of sensory-affective reactions to excessive stimuli. Normally there is a protective mechanism in the sensory affective apparatus against excessive stimuli. Recently a physical-chemical test has been devised to test the threshold of the stimulus barrier (Laufer et al., 1957). Certain hyperkinetic children have been found to have a low threshold, which it has been possible to raise with the aid of amphetamine and also with some tranquilizers, producing bene-ficial effects. Laufer (personal communication) also used ampheta-mine empirically with a group of stutterers. The results were good in those cases where the so-called constitutional factors predomi-nated. The reverse effect—an intensification of the stutter—was noted with the more definitely neurotic group. In the first group there probably were children with a low stimulus threshold. Robert West (1958), one of the group of workers in the field of speech pathology from the ranks of academic psychology, has classified stuttering among the pyknolepsies characterized by a low spasm threshold. It is possible that he and I are talking about the same phenomenon, only I call it low stimulus threshold, which I believe deals with the cause, while he calls it low spasm threshold which describes the consequences. The implications for therapy are different according to whichever view is held.

According to Federn, a similar low threshold of stimulus barrier occurs when the ego boundaries are poorly charged with instinctual energy (see 1952, Ch. 12). This is often the case in the poorly differentiated ego boundaries in the stutterer. Thus a physical defect probably originating in embryonic life may produce the identical effect as faulty ontogenetic development in the form of poor ego differentiation, and vice versa. This is but one of many examples of where it is difficult to distinguish fully the influence of one zone from that of the other.

There is another similarity in the conclusions of the authors who studied the hyperkinetic children and one observer (Karlin, 1947) who attributes stuttering to a lag in myelinization of certain fibers in the central nervous system. It is that the causative factor becomes inoperative or disappears gradually toward the end of adolescence. Eisenson (1958) quotes the neurologist Penfield who thinks of perseveration as a neurological lag. Perhaps it is closer to the facts to state that perseveration is an attempt to bridge the neurological lag, whatever that represents. Delays in maturation of the mental ego organization constitute a counterpart in the psychological development.

Attitudes with respect to the treatment of stuttering are as varied as the ideas concerning its dynamics. Coriat (1933, 1943) made many references to the difficulties in the treatment of stuttering because of the general aspect of the narcissism of the stutterer. However, he did not elaborate on this problem or on ways of dealing with it. Brill (1923), stressing the same obstacle, nevertheless offered a somewhat more hopeful therapeutic outlook by suggesting a few rather simple approaches in dealing with the problem of narcissism. In my own opinion, the outlook for analytic therapy appears brighter than either Coriat or Brill envisaged because of the possibilities I see in exploiting some recent insights arising from advances made in ego psychology.

Finally, what may be said about Freud's attitude regarding the use of psychoanalytic therapy for stuttering? There is no explicit answer to this question in any of his writings, although there are implications that with the passing of time, at least up to a point, he grew more conservative regarding it.

Chapter 3

Freud's Contributions on Stuttering: Their Relation to Some Current Insights*

I am attempting to collate what Freud had written and spoken about the stuttering syndrome; and to review the material in the light of current insights. Surprisingly, what Freud dealt with and touched on clinically and theoretically encompassed nearly all the nodal points of the stuttering syndrome, despite the fact that this clinical material was in many respects quite atypical. On different occasions he discussed aspects of the genesis and dynamics of the symptom; nosology and differential diagnosis; therapy and prognosis. Furthermore, he contributed observations on some of the special features of stuttering such as, for example, its monosymptomatic appearance, and its relation to earlier ego states. Moreover, some of his observations—to borrow a phrase of his own—struck rock bottom, even though they were often stated in terms we might now consider broad.

Freud had only one case history, as far as I know, in which stuttering played an important role.** This is the classical case of Frau Emmy von N., one of the five which composed the "Studies on Hysteria" (Breuer and Freud, 1893–1895).

As may be recalled, he introduced this 40-year-old widow, the

---

*Originally published in the *Journal of the American Psychoanalytic Association*, April 1958, 6(2):326–347.

**Parenthetically, another important Freudian study involved a man, Moses, who is historically recorded as a stutterer. However, Freud regarded the possibility that Moses was not a stutterer, but one whose speech inhibition might be accounted for on the basis that the prophet was an Egyptian unfamiliar with the Hebrew language.

mother of two girls, "as a hysteric [who] could be put into a state of somnambulism with the greatest of ease" (p. 48). The treatment undertaken—catharsis plus suggestion under hypnosis—took place in a nursing home where the patient was seen twice a day. It totaled fifteen weeks within the two years of 1888 to 1890.

Symptoms fell roughly into three groups: a hysterical delirium; facial and neck tics, cramps in the abdomen and legs; and a group of speech disturbances. The latter consisted of a stutter, a tic-like clacking sound, a so-called protective formula consisting of: "Keep still! Don't say anything! Don't touch me!" and an involuntary utterance of her own name which was the same as that of one of her daughters.

My concern here is practically entirely with the third group— her speech. Freud paid considerable attention to the stutter and the clacking. He called the latter a curious sound which defied imitation, adding in a footnote that the clacking "was made up of a number of sounds. Colleagues of mine with sporting experience told me, on hearing it, that its final notes resembled the call of a capercaillie," or woodcock. Strachey (p. 49n) quotes from a book on ornithology: "The sound is a ticking ending with a pop and a hiss." Freud often referred only to the clacking as a tic; at other times he referred to both speech symptoms— the stuttering and the clacking—as tics.

Frau Emmy's stutter was unusual in several ways. For one thing, it occurred in a woman. Stuttering is seen about five to ten times less frequently in women than among men. Furthermore, it seemed to have begun in adult life, which is quite rare, especially without a history of stuttering in childhood. However, stuttering has been observed not uncommonly in the war neuroses in soldiers (Grinker and Spiegel, 1945) with and without a history of childhood stuttering. The factor of trauma as a precipitating event is also very commonly mentioned in the history of the childhood onset. Non-analytic writers (Hahn, 1943, e.g.) also emphasize the traumatogenic tendency in stuttering. I have been similarly impressed with trauma as a precipitating event.

I have also noticed that stutterers in general have a tendency, similar to that of the group of hysterics referred to by Freud in this case history, toward the "primary or instinctual phobias of human beings . . . [which] are established more firmly by traumatic events" (p. 87). These primary phobias include fear of animals, calamitous events in nature, of insanity. At the time that this case history was written, Freud had not yet established the important fact which he later discovered that fantasies may be co-equal in their traumatic effect with external events. The fact is that traumatogenic fantasies relating to the phenomena of primal scene, separation, and castration, appear to be embedded in the clinical material of this case. These fantasies are often elicited in stutterers, and I have found them crucial in contributing to the narcissistic and oral fixations which are so determining for the stutterer. The importance of these fantasies has sometimes been obscured by the emphasis given to Freud's subsequent remark about anal phenomena in stuttering (see Jones, 1955). Freud referred to the stuttering and the clacking as tics of interpolations which intrude upon the voluntary movements of the normal flow of speech without interfering or being mixed with it. Here he drew an interesting parallel with the hysterical delirium which interpolated itself within the normal flow of the conscious state. Furthermore, the two types of interpolation tended to appear simultaneously: the patient stuttering more often during the confusional states. Because these states represented a form of reliving of early traumatic events, and probably even earlier traumatic fantasies, we may say that they constituted the return of early ego states.

So much for the external form of the stuttering and clacking, and some of their superficial associations. What about their content or meaning? Throughout the treatment of Frau Emmy, Freud repeatedly inquired from her, under hypnosis, why she stuttered or clacked whenever she did so more than usually. The application of this comparatively simple procedure resulted in enormously rich clinical material and basic theoretical formulations.

This was Freud's first case in which he used Breuer's method of catharsis. Yet it already contains such psychoanalytic fundamentals as his observation and description of what was later to be called free association, and the first example of the concept of cathexis. There emerged through this process of catharsis somewhere between forty and fifty (there is some overlapping) traumatic events, which are succinctly described. These consist of recent actual events,

memories—both real and screen—dreams, fantasies, and hallucinations. These phenomena contain etiologically significant components of the stuttering disorder which seem to me to be of central
importance, as will be discussed presently.

The pathogenic phenomena visualized by the patient in plastic
form and natural colors are grouped by Freud in a series of three:
early traumata, mainly prepubertal; traumata of the middle and
late teens, causing lasting fright; still later traumata, a series of
surprises. There had been a large number of experiences of
witnessing the illnesses and deaths of her mother, of many siblings
(the patient was the thirteenth of fourteen children of whom only
four survived), and of her husband. The deaths of her mother and
husband were sudden and unexpected. These most significant
experiences were imbued with some aura of unreality, as if the
deceased lived on after the fashion of the frequent theme of being
buried alive. Freud refers to some of these fantasies as hallucinations.
Perhaps they can be more fully comprehended as necrophilic
wishes and fantasies which have the ambivalent aim of retaining
identity with, and yet attaining freedom from, the dead relative. In
one of the hallucinations, Freud's patient saw a dummy sit up in
bed in the home of a friend one year after her mother's death. Frau
Emmy had another component of the necrophilic fantasy—in one
of her dreams she was the passive victim of a vulture.

Her multiple self-representations can be recognized as elements
of the fantasy—body equals phallus—which I was able to discern
bit by bit. Both were contained in a whole series of gruesome stories
about animals: dead rats being stuffed in the mouth and gnawed;
dead animals being thrown at her; a toad under a stone apparently
buried alive. The latter image is overdetermined and seemed to be
related among other things to her mother and cousin being "put
away" in an insane asylum. Insane asylums, besides standing for
losing mother (separation) and losing her power of mind (losing
herself, or being beside herself), also represent losing the power of
speech. She became mute after each hospitalization of a member of
her family. The body-phallus equation accounts for speech or voice
being unconsciously felt as a urethral equivalent, and the loss of
voice or speech as evidence of phallic castration. Thus there is a
series of traumatic—castration—equivalents: separation from love

objects, loss of mental power, loss of power of speech. Her earliest reactions to this trauma were total, but the later ones became gradually more and more circumscribed.

However, the deepest psychopathological root of the speech difficulty goes back to a very early date when a complex of traumatic events affecting the oral zone apparently determined a fixation at that zone. We turn now to these events. She brought up the subject of her cousin. "He was rather queer in the head and his parents had all his teeth pulled out at one sitting" (p. 56). We may wonder to what extent this may be fact, fantasy, or a mixture of both. Freud does not speculate here.

The protective formulae containing elements of avoidance and gratification can be considered symptom-like formations. By contrast, the tonic stuttering and the clacking represent a simpler mechanism. One is the result of an attempt at inhibition or mutism, and the other, a breakthrough of sounds or the failure of the inhibition. In other words, each represents one half of the symptom isolated from the other.

As already mentioned, Freud repeatedly inquired into the onset and causes of the stutter.

Not infrequently when the patient did not recall a fact Freud asked her to remember it under hypnosis. On one occasion he asked her to remember the origin of the stuttering at the next hypnotic session. This she did "without any further reflection but in great agitation and with spastic impediments in her speech. 'How the horses bolted once with the children in the carriage; and how another time I was driving through the forest with the children in a thunderstorm and a tree just in front of the horses was struck by lightning and the horses shied, and I thought: "You must keep quite still now, or your screaming will frighten the horses even more and the coachman won't be able to hold them in at all." It came on from that moment'" (p. 58). She further said that the stutter began immediately after the first of these occasions but disappeared shortly afterward, and then recurred and remained after the second, similar occasion.

Freud writes that the patient's clacking sound, always referred to as a tic or ticlike sound, went back, like the earlier tonic stutter, to similar precipitating causes and had an analogous mechanism. The clacking sound was precipitated at "a time when she was sitting by the bedside of her younger daughter who was very ill, and had wanted to keep absolutely quiet" (p. 54). Later on, the clacking came on whenever she was apprehensive or frightened.

In his discussion of the various symptoms, Freud classifies those relating to the patient's speech among the phobias and abulias, the latter two being causally related. As an example of a phobia—a term used here synonymously with fear—he mentions her fear of thunderstorms, which corresponds to the primary or instinctive fears of human beings, "and especially of neuropaths." He then adds: "But these phobias too were established more firmly by traumatic events" (p. 87). As regards the more specific phobias which are accounted for by particular events, Freud writes: "In my opinion, however, all these psychical factors, though they may account for the *choice* of these phobias, cannot explain their *persistence*" (p. 88). For the latter he finds it necessary to adduce a *neurotic* factor in the sense of what he later termed the "actual neuroses." Freud thus establishes a sequence: instinctive fears— their activation by traumata—their maintenance by a neurotic factor which is in essence the patient's massive sexual repression.

It is obvious that the precipitating cause of both the stutter and the sound tic consists of the patient's fear of uttering a sound or making a noise. In the one case, the sound might have caused the horses to run wild and thus possibly hurt the children; and in the other, it might have caused the harmful wakening of the sick child who had at last fallen asleep.

All of the four related speech symptoms, collectively classed as ticlike movements, are based on a general mechanism which Freud designates as, "the putting into effect of antithetic ideas," which are obviously painful and fearsome. In the case of the tonic stutter, there is an attempt to block ideas that are opposite in nature to those which the conscious will aims to express. The clacking sounds, on the one hand, represent the result of an *unsuccessful* blocking and the emergence of

> . . . a succession of sounds which are convulsively emitted and separated by pauses and which could best be likened to clacking. It appears a conflict had occurred between her intention and the antithetic idea (the counter-will) and that this gave the *tic* its discontinuous character

and confined the antithetic idea to paths other than the habitual ones for innervating the muscular apparatus of speech.

The exciting cause—the antithetic idea—was essentially similar in both manifestations. In the "peculiar stammer was the attempted convulsive inhibition of the organs of speech which was made into a symbol of the event for her memory, while in the tic it was the outcome of the final innervation—the exclamation."

Thus the speech of Frau Emmy was affected in a threefold manner: by attempted tonic spasms (inhibition); by a breakthrough of a peculiar involuntary sound marking the failure of inhibition; and by the involuntary uttering of words called protective formulae, more closely approximating symptom formation. Freud attempts to elucidate on only the first two—the stuttering and the clacking—by means of the mechanism "of the putting into effect of feared antithetic ideas."

In the light of our understanding today, the feared antithetic idea of Frau Emmy as it relates etiologically to the stuttering and the clacking seems now to be analyzable, the abundant clinical material cited by Freud substantiating such analysis. It is obvious that there is an inherent connection, amounting to an essential identity, between Frau Emmy's repressed and feared ideas or wishes from the past and the feared events which she described as precipitating the stutter and the clacking. The common thought is that a child might be harmed or killed. It is also apparent that both the image of "a child" and the idea of "being harmed or killed" have multiple meanings.

First, I will discuss the idea of being harmed or killed. The dangerous milieu is one of lightning amidst loud noise. The deadly agency is a compound of sound—a voice, or a thunder, of runaway horses, and of lightning striking (consuming) a tree. Voice, tree, and horses are phallic images; sounding, running, consuming denote phallic and oral destructiveness. Furthermore, one of the patient's defensive formulae, "keep still," is directed against animal shapes which would attack if anyone moved. She is likewise afraid to interrupt the frightening thoughts. She seems fearful and fascinated. This is strongly suggestive of a compulsion to repeat a traumatic event or fantasy. It doubtless belongs, as do the other elements just mentioned, to the primal scene.

Now, in the second place, what about the object in this series of traumatic events and fantasies? It is manifestly, first of all, Frau Emmy's real child. But simultaneously it is also Frau Emmy herself as a child, whose unconscious memories threaten to return as a result of her identification with her child who is now facing similar traumatic events.

In the first series—the early memories—the siblings who died and the patient herself were young children. Here the specific images of "children" were real. The concepts of "dying" were experienced as real and by identification. However, in the second and third series—lasting frights and surprises—we find, in addition, fears of separation, castration, and incorporation. The image of the "child" that is being harmed in these traumatizing experiences refers to the child-phallus equation, also to the equation of the whole body as phallus. The nature of the harm as it is portrayed in the reaction is therefore separation, castration, and death.

Freud (1900–1901) called attention to the fact that to the dreamer speech represents life whereas muteness represents death; and that a child represents the phallus. That the entire body may be symbolized by the phallus has been noted by Ferenczi (1917, 1928), Abraham (1924), and Tausk (1934). Lewin (1933) found the body-phallus fantasy as the self-image in two female stutters (see Ch. 2). At approximately the same time, Bunker (1934) called attention to the unconscious identity of the voice and the female phallus.

From my own experience, which included the analyses of stutterers, parents of stutterers, and the children of stutterers, I discovered the following continuum. From the mothers I learned that they identify themselves with the breast and imaginary phallus of their mothers as well as with the phallus of their fathers. Furthermore, they regard their stuttering child as their own ablated breast-phallus and repeat the process of appersonation with it. In analyzing the stutterer I found that he has a similar part-object self-image. In turn, he tends to appersonate his child, as he was appersonated by his mother, in terms of the breast-phallic image. In my experience, the symbiotic need and its converse—separation anxiety—as expressed through the body-phallus fantasy occur so uniformly that they strike me as unique in the genesis of stuttering.

They seem unlike similar needs or anxiety in other disorders, qualitatively, quantitatively, or both. I believe they determine an accentuated orality with fluctuating active and passive aims.

We return now to some genetic factors in the case of Frau Emmy. The actual references to her parents are meager but suggestive. Freud remarks that "she was brought up carefully but under strict discipline by an overenergetic and severe mother" (p. 49). The patient herself speaks of "being as one" with her father by identifying her own digestive idiosyncrasies with his. From Freud's description of the personality of his patient, she appears also to have been rather overenergetic and masculine. Without comment, he quotes her reason for not marrying again, namely, her distrust of the intentions of her suitors who might be after her fortune, which she is determined to guard carefully on behalf of her daughters. This is quite at variance with an actual appeal made to Freud by one of the daughters when she was grown, married, and had become a doctor. She complained that her mother had refused her any share of the inheritance. This contradiction can be explained by Frau Emmy's ambivalent attitude toward her inheritance, which is an anal-phallic gift from her parents, if not exclusively from her father.

Frau Emmy was an anxious mother. She often feared calamities such as mental illnesses—"losing one's mind"—befalling her children; also fatal accidents, such as might be caused by the falling of the elevator in the pension where they lived. Misfortunes such as these further suggest ideas of separation and castration. Apparently her children were to her anal-phallic gifts analogous to the worldly ones. In the case of the latter the conflict was between retention and separation. But what was it about in relation to her children? They were experienced as her phallic part-selves, poorly integrated with her other self-representations and tending to be readily externalized. Thus, the births of the children and the various phases of their nurturing and differentiating must have been experienced by the mother as hostile separations, disrupting her narcissistic ideal self-image. The need to reinstate this ideal image which was always on the verge, or seemingly in process, of disintegration led to deep wishes to eat, to reincorporate the children. It is this orally aggressive wish which became the repressed painful antithetic idea.

The external events, already described, which helped precipitate the stuttering and the clacking were so strikingly similar to the repressed "antithetic idea" that it was as if the repressed had actually returned to consciousness. The results were an anxiety signal and the instituting of defensive measures in the form of inhibitions in Frau Emmy's speech. The inhibitions were not complete; they allowed an occasional breakthrough of a sound largely distorted by the defensive struggle.

My own observations suggest that the dominant instinctual fixation is oral passivity plus a reactive accentuation of oral aggression. The need to inhibit both expressions through speech simultaneously with the wish to express them produces the conflict that is reflected in the stutter. Stated in structural terms, the conflict is between the emerging ego state which uses speech realistically and as sublimation and the same ego regressing to states of pre-ego whose dominant aim is to re-establish or maintain the mother-child identity by using the speech apparatus, the mouth, in accordance with its primary function.

Was Freud intuitively aware of the fundamental oral conflict underlying Frau Emmy's speech difficulties? The possibility suggests itself because he illustrated the concept of contrasting ideas or "counter-will" by referring to a case he had reported on earlier (Freud, 1893). This was a woman who, each time she gave birth—it happened twice—got sick over the struggle to nurse her child against her neurotic inability to do so, a classical post-partum oral conflict. Here again, Freud did not analyze the meaning of her "counter-will," but only pointed to the fact of her physical exhaustion, which facilitated the emergence of the repressed wish.

In summary, the repressed antithetical idea of Frau Emmy which affected her speech is a compound of several related ones. First, there is the most important predisposing one: repression of the oedipal wish ending in total repression of her sexuality, as alluded to by Freud. Second, to maintain this massive repression of genital libido plus the associated aggression, additional defenses were instituted by regression to phallic, anal, but especially oral libidinal phases. If we turn now from the instinctual to the structural point of view, we may say the antithetical idea was imbedded in the ego domain following regression from object libido. The conflict was between integration of the narcissistic components on the magical level of the mother-child appersonation and the splitting up of the appersonation by the separation and externalization of the child-phallus component—in other words, the emergence of object libido. This threat of separation activated aggressive reincorporative and retentive, i.e., "restitutive" oral drives, which constituted the antithetical idea.

Speech lends itself as the vehicle for expression of all the instinctual drives, and, inasmuch as, in the unconscious, to express a wish by means of thoughts and words is equivalent to a literal living out of such a wish, thoughts and speech are highly cathected with libidinal and aggressive energy in their various forms of expression. Nevertheless, the instinctual forms of expression exert a predominant claim upon the function of speech. Various reasons for this fact have already been cited. We must not omit the most obvious, namely, that speech actually exploits the physical oral apparatus since it has none of its own. Inasmuch as speech can and does subserve all of the partial drives, in sublimated forms, it is frequently subject to distortion by formation of symptoms when these drives are involved in conflicts. The conflict situations which most often affect these drives and produce symptoms are to be found especially in the phenomena of the primal scene, separation, castration, and the oedipal situation.

A significant aspect of stuttering, one which is in large measure responsible for its relative intractibility, is that it frequently presents itself, especially in adults, as a *monosymptomatic* disorder. Even when it is not monosymptomatic, as in the case of Frau Emmy, the chronic stutter is highly overdetermined, the determinants building up in the manner of a chain of phobic associations. Freud not only took notice of these facts, but also offered an explanation.

It was based in part on Frau Emmy's self-observations, which Freud accepted, and in part on his own findings in the case of Elizabeth von R., another of the patients in the "Studies on Hysteria" who suffered from astasia-abasia. The two cases are analogous in that both involve physical automatisms learned very early in life and approximately during the same period. Frau Emmy, in offering an explanation for the incompleteness of the therapeutic success with her speech symptoms, said that "she had got into the habit of stammering and clacking *whenever* she was frightened, so that in the end the symptoms had come to be attached not solely to the initial traumas but to a long chain of memories associated with them." Freud added that this was in accordance with the mechanism of monosymptomatic hysteria which he observed in Fraulein Elizabeth von R. In brief, in this patient, every fresh theme which had a pathogenic effect produced: (a) a new painful area in her legs in extension from the previous one; (b) constantly accumulated cathexis of the various functions of the legs linking these functions with her feelings of pain; (c) the painful thoughts found a symbolic expression through her physical suffering.

Later studies of the monosymptomatic neurosis by other analysts (Gerard, 1947; Lieberman, 1924) have stressed early traumatic experiences inhibiting natural muscular responses; the mechanisms of repetition compulsion and isolation; narcissistic hurts from childhood illnesses; and the use of the symptom as a magical gesture denoting wishes from and a threat toward the parents. With the possible exception of the last factor, all the rest appear to be encompassed in Freud's observations.

In summary, though Freud touched on many aspects of stuttering, his contributions fall into two main categories. One is the case report of Frau Emmy von N., which abounds in uniquely rich clinical observations. The theoretical concern in this case, however, is practically exhausted by ramifications of the general phenomenon of conversion. The other category is theoretical only, composed of several dynamic and nosologic formulations. Of these, perhaps none has attained greater prominence than one factor—that of instinctual regression, or, as Freud put it, concretely, the fact that stutterers project upon the oral apparatus the instinctual conflicts of the anal zone. However, it is my contention that, while not detracting from the validity of projection upward of anal material, there are other, deeper, and more significant dynamic factors in stuttering; furthermore, these other factors also may, with current insights, be found documented in the clinical material on Frau Emmy, as well as in implications in Freud's discussion of Federn's paper on asthma. These factors consist first of all of determining fixations within narcissistic-oral developmental levels. In the second place, as a result of the emphasis upon the pregenital nature of the conversion, the most significant role of the unresolved oedipal conflict as a constant dynamic factor in maintaining the regression and the symptom has perhaps not been assigned its proper weight. In the case of Frau Emmy, Freud stresses the fact of the maintenance of the neurosis by the patient's total repression of her sexuality, although the report antedates his discovery of the Oedipus conflict. Lastly, in relation to the controversy about the symptom serving predominantly or exclusively impulse or defense—in other words, whether it represents perversion or neurosis—I may say the following: In the first place, Freud himself stated that at the point of organ fixation hysteria approaches the perversions. However, he stressed that the pregenital conversions also differ from hysteria in regard to the problem of narcissism. It may then be said that the sharp distinction between neuroses and perversions relates mainly to the classical transference neuroses. When we consider narcissistic or ego-defect neuroses, especially from the standpoint of aggressive drives, the sharpness of the distinction is blurred, so that these disorders partake, especially as regards the structure of the ego, of attributes of both.

Chapter 4

Theoretical Considerations

In his first year of life, the child's principal relationship to the world is by way of his mouth. The mouth not only serves his nutrition, but may be considered the master organ that sets off and stimulates other functions—especially respiration and neurosensory integration. The tactile sensations in the mouth set off by sucking produce a sense of well-being by discharge of tension inherent in the mouth musculature. In addition, because of the increased oxygen flow to the brain resulting from nursing and being held, there is a reflex stimulation of the gastrointestinal tract, the respiratory tract, and the central nervous system. Other effects of nursing are rest and relaxation, which are indispensable for the development of the infant's ego.

We can only infer what the infant's subjective state is before he begins to speak. All indications point to the infant's feeling a oneness with the mother and her breast—the infant is in a state of biopsychologic symbiosis. Nursing and satiety produce pleasure, and hunger produces pain. Pleasure and satiety produce a feeling of omnipotence; hunger and pain, a state of shock (severe regression, partial death). In this context food acquires magical power identical with the mother and the outside world. The mother is considered as a kind of detachable organ that functions only as the executor of the will of the child, having magical or omnipotent powers for satisfaction (Ferenczi, 1913).

Gradually the child develops an awareness of a gulf existing between him and the mother—a landmark in the emergence of the sense of self. But for a relatively long time the emerging self is still cushioned against the shocking feeling of being all alone by images of the blissful state of fusion. As the ego evolves out of the instinctual energy release, it stimulates other organs, such as the eyes, ears, skin, and central nervous system, into pleasurable sensory activity resulting in further growth of the ego.

During this earliest state of narcissism the mouth is the magical or animistic organ, and food represents mother and infant (Freud, 1914). Subjectively, relationships with other individuals have reality only if they can be similarly controlled by incorporation, assimilation, and identification with the infant. Since interpersonal relationships are nonexistent, speech even as inarticulate sound does not exist. Only incorporation by way of the mouth has validity, and the earliest precursors of speech at this time—babbling and crying—have only narcissistic and autoerotic meanings.

By the second year, the child begins to be disciplined increasingly, that is to say, deprived of oral satisfactions through weaning from the breast and from other tactile satisfactions. This is a critical time, but the child is sustained, first, by the confidence gained from the experience of steady oral indulgence and, second, by the emergence of new pleasure-giving organs—the eyes, the ears, and the hands. The grasping and holding acts originate from nursing by substitution of "distance receptors" for "mediate receptors."

Shortly after weaning from breast and bottle comes the second major crisis—the discipline and deprivations of bowel and bladder training. Attention is focused on another zone of instinctual gratification—the anus. Hitherto enjoyed without voluntary control, the function of elimination has now to be controlled consciously. At first the child is apprehensive because he has to postpone the release of tension and because his mother seems to be determined to rob him of something. If all has gone well in his development hitherto, we may suppose that the child successfully emerges from this critical period. When he does, he learns that instinctual gratification is not lost by postponement. (Neither is it lost by sublimation of coprophilia into love for painting, sculpturing, etc.) But the most important gains from this phase of development are in the realm of the ego, at the expense of dependence upon and identification with mother. Perhaps for the first time the child is struck with the fact that he has a will of his own, that he can use it to initiate an act, that, though subject to parental pressures, he and not they has complete control of this function. This period in the life of the child is further marked by rapid spurts in intellectual growth.

Mouth and anus are organically connected; so are the functions of incorporation, on the one hand, and of retention and elimination, on the other. By the same token, the archaic conceptions of power and control attached to the mouth still linger about the anus, but with one important difference—that at the anal phase the power stems not from animistic fusion or identification with the mother or mother world, but from an interplay of magical strengths between powerful ego and powerful figures in the environment. Elimination of feces symbolizes this power. The speech function at this stage is for the first time an instrument of the personality of the child as distinct from the mother. The need is still to cling to her, but now articulate speech is used as an instrument of control on a more realistic basis.

The genital stage concerns the pathology of stuttering less than the earlier phases. The sense of self is now more fully developed, and object relationships are less burdened by archaic animistic conceptions. Love as it develops for the parents at this stage is now transferred to other individuals in the form of affectionate social feelings. The sense of reality about people and the world is established. Speech now becomes an instrument of interpersonal relationships, expression ideas and feelings on a more realistic level.

While some stuttering children have attained this normal attitude, i.e., the genital stage of development, the large majority have not. They have been arrested at the oral stage. In essence this means that although they are exposed to the later normalizing stimuli and seemingly act and feel normally, the "unfinished business" of the oral phase remains active in the unconscious and radially distorts the conceptions of self and of others, and their emotions and behavior.

Why the Oral Arrest?

The basic trauma in stutterers is the faulty dissolution of the primary identification with the mother. The mother, because of her own psychological problems, has not provided adequately for the child. Ribble (1941) has described the stimulus hunger that results from inadequate mothering. The mothers of stutterers alternately cling to and reject their infants. The baby's separation from the mother apparantly begins prematurely and in consequence is also delayed. Because the infant deals with it by means of a primary repression, before speech and ego development, it is perhaps never quite possible to re-experience it fully in therapy and completely overcome it. The most important aspect of this trauma is the poor management of sucking through poor holding, improper rhythm, and inadequate volume. Relatively less important, but in itself very significant, is premature training of the function of elimination, the effect of which is equivalent to separation from the mother.

The infantile trauma produces motor and psychic effects. The motor effects appear before the psychic and in a way mutely express them in the pantomime language of patterns of muscle tension. These remain throughout life, alongside the psychic reactions that become manifest in the second quarter of the first year. Probably the most potent psychic reaction to the trauma is anxiety and its essential meaning is reaction to the danger of loss of mother. The ego, hemmed in by anxiety arising from the increasing tension of inner hunger, is in a state of arrest. It never completes its differentiation from mother and her breast, so that the boundaries of self and others remain hazy. The symbiotic fusion remains. Any push in the direction of self-differentiation results in marked anxiety with increased clinging. A large portion of the subjective state of magical being and thinking—primary narcissism—remains fixed. All objects are regarded as magical omnipotent mothers from whom one is inseparable. The technique of relationship consists of wishes that have omnipotent properties, and mother as their private executive is believed to know them even before they are articulated. Or else the articulated words have the same magical attributes. If there is any hitch in the process of fulfillment, the child resorts to tantrums or to acts of ingratiation or appeasement. The mouth retains its major function of clinging to objects—animate as well as inanimate. The differentiated forms of oral activity—biting, chewing, smiling, crying, and vocalization—maintain the intensity and energy of the original sucking.

It is the anxiety that is now responsible for a most significant element in this entire picture, namely, aggression. Whether this aggressiveness represents retaliation against a hostile environment or the stirring up of deep innate regressive forces destructive to the ego when the going is too hard, or both, is moot. From the practical standpoint, however, the aggression is of transcendent importance because it lends an ambivalent quality to the entire magical structure. The child, now conscious of mother as having magical powers for good and evil, attributes to himself, through identification with her, omnipotent powers for construction and destruction. The child's aggressions cannot be expressed openly for fear of provoking the wrath of the powerful parent. This leads to withdrawal. But his helplessness leads him to get close again to the good image of the parent, only to feel repelled again by fear of mutual aggression. The result is harmful in a twofold way: relationships become oscillating, and there is estrangement from the real feelings of the self because they become dangerous and are repressed.

The profound craving for oral dependence on the mother, subjectively felt as omnipotence, is regarded by the ego as a threat to its integrity or very life. It rightly regards it as an oral aggression upon itself and reacts by wishes to retaliate in kind. Besides, the ego is itself identified with the aggressor (Anna Freud, 1936). When this psychic ambivalence is viewed from the standpoint of its somatic expression (conversion), we see that speech and respiration, which "take in" the environment, express this oral dependence and oral aggression. Since both threaten the ego, resistances are set up against both. The conflict of whether or not to depend, whether or not to be aggressive, is equivalent to the conflict of whether or not to speak. Hence the speech becomes halting, its smooth flow interrupted by tonic and clonic spasms.

The study of stutterers and their family backgrounds indicates that after the neurosis is established it continues to maintain itself by its own intrapsychic momentum and the pathogenic influence of the mother continues unabatedly active. That activity did not stem merely and primarily from such strong feelings as rejection, a mixture of love and hate, and so on. These were observed, to be sure, although they were often accompanied by much genuine affection. More fundamentally, the activity stemmed from an anxious incapacity of the mother to separate from the child, whom she unconsciously felt to be an integral part of her own body—an organ, as it were. It is necessary, therefore, to understand the personality of the mother since she is the dominant parent in the first year of the child's life, the mother-child relationship (including the important place of the father in the family picture), and the mother's unique attitude toward speech. These three phenomena are bound together like mathematical functions.

The Mother of the Stutterer

To the world at large, the mother usually gives a good general impression: she is presentable, responsible, and seems to be emotionally warm. Outside her relationships to her child and secondarily to her husband, which present problems, she seems to have good control of her life situation. Regarding her stuttering child, one notes at once her great activity in seeking help, and the unmistakable fact that she showers much affection on him. Later it becomes evident that the relationship is a "sticky" one, for she invests more attention in him, also more concern, preoccupation, possessiveness, and control than perhaps in all the rest of the members of the family. Regardless of the boy's age, he occupies first place in her life. An example of this tenacious tie of the mother to the child is the frequency of the mother's discontinuation of treatment of the child after it has got well under way, unless in the original treatment plan proper attention is given the mother, simultaneously with or prior to the child's treatment. The maternal affect most commonly shown is great anxiety centered around the child's speech, his general behavior, his masturbation, his school or social life. Below the surface, envy, disappointment, and hostility are also found.

In most of the spheres of her own life the mother is aware of insecurity. She also has emotional, behavioral, and sexual inhibitions, of which she is mostly unaware. She is likewise unaware that she is burdened by separation fears, guilt, and aggression. Her life history frequently reveals that she suffered from masochistic dependence on her own mother who, though she too might have been infantile in some ways, appeared to have a stronger character than the mother herself. Both mother and grandmother idealized active and aggressive people, usually personified in some male relative of theirs, perhaps a nephew or a grandfather. Later idealization referred primarily to an image of their ego ideal. Thus, the children—the stutterer and his mother (as a child)—in the lives of their respective mothers, witnessed oscillation between extremes of weakness and strength. The "strength" took the form either of futile strivings toward an ego ideal or of impotent rage at failure to attain it. Generally, the mother's behavior was impressed upon the child as genuine strength. The image of the mother as a powerful figure was maintained for a very long time. Her weaknesses, on the other hand, were recognized only at a much later age.

Psychosexually, the mother has a poorly differentiated sense of self—part child, part tomboy, part wife-husband. Penis envy or competitiveness with males is a frequent component, as is the history of being in love with a masculine type of man and marrying another, weaker type. The marriage may generally be characterized as sadomasochistic, propelled mainly by a need to control or by a sense of duty, and little by pleasurable pursuits.

In the early days of psychoanalysis the mother would have been diagnosed as a hysteric: she is anxious, her object-directed libido is repressed, and her object choice is bisexually balanced. However, in the light of our more recent knowledge of the development of the ego, narcissism, and aggression, she can be seen in clearer perspective. We can now recognize that her disturbed object relations are to a considerable extent not genuine object relations. Instead, love objects represent to her narcissistic objects—self-images, idealized and/or degraded.

Since this fact is very close to the heart of the problem, we must define narcissistic objects. To do so, we have to digress somewhat into early ego development. Freud called the primary phase of the ego organization the pleasure-ego of the baby. The self-image of this preverbal period of life, reconstructed from many pieces of evidence, is that of a breast. It merges with or separates from the maternal body, thus multiplying the number of self-images. Furthermore, this sense of oneness flowing from the image of fusion with the mother is felt as a pleasurable, omnipotent, inexhaustible, suprahuman reservoir of security. This highly charged picture has been called the narcissistic ego-ideal (Freud, 1914). When the child's early security is seriously impaired, this mystical union is felt to be broken into its various component parts: breast, and later, phallus, separated from the idealized body, and the latter damaged as a result of the separations. These separated elements are then perceived as unattractive, impotent, yet aggressively charged, and the aim is to regain the former state of union.

All this is seen more clearly when the mother is studied analytically in relation to her separation anxieties—from her own mother and later from the child—and her wish for a return to the early state of symbiosis. Now, the fact is that this state of oneness as it is felt and visualized is the norm at a very early stage of ego development. Under certain adverse conditions unusually strong memories of this magical, ideal ego state are retained, as well as memories of fears of a tendency to split into the component parts. At a later phase of ego growth a more highly developed defensive reaction appears—the process of identification. The retention of the earlier, archaic self-images has been aptly termed identification with the aggressor (Anna Freud, 1936) and the loss of sense of self, accompanied by an emotional impoverishment. This tendency to shift from a self-image of an ideal ego to one of a separate part results in ambivalence, aggressiveness, and exhibitionism. The latter is a magical gesture serving as a plea to be reincorporated to assuage the separation anxiety and to lessen the inner aggressiveness.

What are these adverse conditions? In the analyses of a group of mothers of stutterers I invariably found disappointment in their own fathers and a characteristically strong tie to their own mothers or what their mothers stood for. Attempts at separation from their mothers or from their mental representations, that is, certain traits and attitudes representing them, always produced intense anxiety. As a consequence they never succeeded in shaking the strong ambivalent identification they had with both parents, but especially with the mother. At a later date certain aspects of these ideal or hostile self-images were projected upon their husbands and stuttering children. A composite picture of the mothers of these women is that of an inwardly dependent and anxious woman, subject to stubbornness and emotional outbursts into verbal barrages, though outwardly giving the appearance of activity and strength. As already mentioned, she is outspoken in her idealization of power and control, generally symbolized by masculine exhibitionistic images patterned after some male member of her own family. The early traumatic maternal relationship—between the mother and the grandmother of the stuttering child—is not to be viewed as a single, sharply defined event such as weaning from the breast, but something that may be described teleologically as a lack of that fundamental, steady, affective support essential for the emotional maturation of a child. The total effect on the mother of the stutterer is a disturbance of her basic trust in her external environment and in herself, resulting in retardation in ego development. The most striking consequences in her total personality include denial of her femininity, great reduction of spontaneous activity expressed through multiple inhibitions, and repression of large quantities of rage and defiance. Another crucial result is that she ties up her husband and child with her own phallic and castrated self-images, which she projects upon both of them. The husband stands for her passive self or for her own mother. Thus, she feels he is incapable of adequate or consistent love or that he represents her own phallic ideal self. In the latter case she envies him when he is successful or mocks him when he is not. In brief, the mother's marital relationship is one of identification and projection.

The Mother-Child Relationship

The history of the mother's relationship to her child showed that the child, too, represented the mother's self-images. Pregnancy, to her, meant her own transformation into the ideal phallic mother, complete and powerful, and a denial of separation from this mother figure. It also denied femininity, which was despised as synonymous with passivity, exposing her to hurts and mutilation. Labor of childbirth was often dramatically described as a painful experience of being dismembered. Giving birth led to a redistribution of self-images by a projection upon the child of her passive, inadequate, hated self-image and also of her idealized, narcissistic, phallic self-image. Which of these images was accentuated depended in many cases upon the sex of the child or its physical resemblance to real or idealized individuals significant in the mother's life.

Feeding difficulties, invariably traceable to a hesitant or uniquely ambivalent attitude on the part of the mother, were almost always present during the first year of the child's life. Closer scrutiny revealed the special characteristics of the ambivalence: alternations of aggressive feeding gestures with sudden withholding, both accompanied by anxiety. One might call this mother a "stuttering" feeder, stamping the pattern of hesitation primarily upon the oral musculature, and secondarily upon the respiratory musculature, of the child. This pattern reappeared in the child when the same organ systems later had to be adapted for the function of speech. Here we see the first instance of characteristic maternal behavior following the mother's projection upon the child of her own contradictory self-images. In other words, the mother fluctuated between a wish to feed the child and make it independent, and a wish to reincorporate the child and thus to regain the image of her perfect or ideal self, which she had in pregnancy. One mother stated that her nursing difficulties stemmed from a fear that the child would eat her up. This was a projection of her own wishes, and an identification with the child's own fantasies—to eat up and to be eaten. What was striking was the sense of realness with which the fear existed in the mother's mind. Nursing was acted out as a repetitive series of aggressive feeding and sudden weaning acts, reaching its climax in the final weaning from breast or bottle. The histories of the children showed that they mimicked the maternal fears. Thus, in many stutterers mother and child were found to simulate and stimulate each other's fantasies.

Various happenings in the child's life, such as birth, nursing, and onset of speech were felt by the mother as anxious experiences, with a special quality compounded of both separation and clutching. Also the child's taking control of his own locomotion, elimination, the development of his will in its negative and positive aspects, and of his intellect—all these landmarks of his ego development—were felt by the mother to be provocative acts of moving away from her. They represented images of acts of biting into and out of the idealized mother-child unity.

What was the effect upon the growing child of such a series of spoken and unspoken signs of anxiety on the part of the mother, in response to the onset of each successive stage in his own ego development? It was apt to be the emergence, at each stage, of parallel fearful and hesitant attitudes, later augmented by feelings of guilt and pent-up aggression. It follows logically, and could be observed clinically, that the psychopathology of the stutterer in essence is based upon inadequate development of certain of his own executant, reality oriented ego functions. Paradoxically, it sometimes seemed that the young stutterer, like the compulsive neurotic, had a precocious ego development, but this ego development generally referred to certain perceptive intellectual abilities, unmatched by similar development in reality testing and in the capacity to bear frustrations.

The Mother's Archaic Conceptions of Speech

It is obvious that speech makes use of the organs of the oral apparatus—the lips, mouth, pharynx, and so on—which are the first organs of contact of the infant with the mother. It has been pointed out that, from this first contact, anxiety and ambivalence characterized the mother's feelings and behavior. She behaved as if she were anxious about what she and the extension of herself, her child, might do with their oral apparatus. At the onset of the child's speech the anxiety, though not its meaning, became more overt. When a child begins to speak toward the end of the second year, it is quite normal for him to repeat the first syllable. These normal iterations were envisaged by his mother as stuttering, and its "dire" consequence on the child's personality was soon established in her mind. This fear represented an apprehension that self-expression on the part of the child was an oral aggression upon her, the mother, with the aim of separation. Paradoxically, the possibility that the child might express passive or nursing wishes was also feared.

During this early stage of the child's learning to speak, the mother often compared the child with her husband or her brother, who frequently actually was a stutterer. Consequently the child, whose oral apparatus had already been impressed with hesitations from his nursing experience, sensed that to his mother speech was overladen with forbidden content—that speech itself was in fact something of a forbidden object. The mother was unusually speech conscious; speech for her had retained its archaic quality of possessing special magical power, either in aggressive acts or passive wishes. Speech, which is a self-revealing, symbolic expression of thinking and feeling ordinarily experienced as a substitute for action, was felt by the mother more nearly as an action than as a symbol. Good speech was highly overvalued by the mother and feared for the same irrational reasons. Speech became the tool of her own oral dependent needs and of her twofold identifications with passive and with aggressive images. By the feeling of oneness, the stuttering child became the instrument of expression for her own aims which were at once passive and aggressive. The stutter, then, represents a composite: a partially unsuccessful attempt to block speech and an exhibitionistic outcropping of it. As already mentioned, speech is felt as aggressive and masochistic acts. It is perfectly consistent in the unconscious mind to have a wish to eat and to be eaten up simultaneously, since the aim is to become one with the other person. Active and passive methods thus become confluent and interchangeable.

We might say that the stutterer is his mother's spokesman. Because the child is part of her, she fears that in his speech he may divulge many of her ambivalences, including pent-up rage and defiance. She begins to fear his speech, which uses the oral apparatus already conditioned to hesitation by her ambivalent feeding of him. Her wish to help him develop into an idealized, powerful individual by separating and building up his own self, along with more or less subtle proddings toward active, perfectionistic goals, is countered by an opposing wish not to have him develop and separate from her, expressed in her attempts to seduce him into helplessness. Indeed, she fears both her wish to feed and free him and her wish to reincorporate and bind him. He in turn senses both fears, which become welded to the functioning of his oral apparatus and constitute the major determinant for the stutter.

The Role of the Father and the Total Family Problem

The father also contributed to both the development and maintenance of the stuttering disorder. His contribution to its development was significant to the degree that he was in flight from his proper relationship to his wife. His contribution to the maintenance of the disorder depended upon the degree of his involvement as a father figure with the stuttering child. Thus, the father might be lacking in a twofold way. Realistically, he was generally in flight from playing a consistent and meaningful role. It can readily be recognized that this flight from the child resembled his withdrawal from his proper marital role. In our experience, when the father did take a consistent and active interest in the stuttering child the prognosis was invariably more favorable. Furthermore, the home situation frequently appeared paradoxical. Articulated strife and contention between the parents often produced relatively less disturbance in the children and a better prognosis than when the atmosphere was all quiet. Often this was the quiet of fear and resignation on the part of one parent to the domination of the other. Here the child incessantly had to witness the same unmitigated control under which he himself suffered.

On the other hand, the quiet of mutual parental acceptance was often based on mutual acceptance of each other's neurotic ties. This usually meant an exchange of normal roles between parents, and led to confusion of identity in the child. Also, a protesting mother or father was therapeutically more reachable than a frightened, resigned, or guilt-imbued parent. A neurotic parental combination which led to a united front often exluded the child from real closeness to either one. While there was no doubt that the primary pathogenic relationship was between mother and child, there was always the possibility that the father could mitigate the mother's infantile traits and assist in the emotional development of his wife. In the same way he could also help the child. Thus, the pathogenesis of stuttering, like its therapy, was shown to be a total family problem.

Remaining Problems

Perhaps at this point it is well to scrutinize some unsolved problems related to stuttering. It has been said that psychoanalysis is basically a labor of search rather than research. It is part of the broad process of empirical observation. Each patient is an experiment of nature rather than a controlled experiment of the laboratory. The rigid requirements of the psychoanalytic hour and the prior analysis of the analyst—the observer—are attempts, as far as is humanly possible, to control the milieu of the observational experiment so as to keep it free from interference with the essence of what is observed. As it has its own range of efficacy, psychoanalysis also has its own limits. It is not geared for fine quantitative evaluation, for example. But in the detailed study of ego disturbances there is a place for research in the laboratory by means of the controlled experiment. However, the vaunted accuracy of such an experiment is valid only within its own context. Its techniques have limits as has its scope. The statistical, questionnaire, etc., methodologies can also misinform when applied to scopes that are too broad or complex for their application.

Nevertheless, there are problems in speech pathology wherein the searchers can turn to the researchers for further elaboration. For example, we need to know more about the natural history of stuttering. Regarding its course of development we know roughly the statistical drop in incidence from childhood to adult life. But we are uncertain about a number of phenomena. For example, does the stutter disappear symptomatically only, or is there also an underlying characterological change? A good many fathers of stutterers I see who have a memory or a history of stuttering in childhood and who regard themselves as "free" of it now, I regard as "cryptic stutterers" with respect to both their speech fluency and personality. Again, on several occasions I have read clinical papers by colleagues about two patients whom I have recognized to be stutterers. This fact was not mentioned in these papers. On inquiry I learned that they did stutter, but neither complained about it nor got involved with it in therapy. We need more information about this group.

Another great need is to resolve the confusion about the problem of therapy. Some analysts recommend analysis or analytically oriented psychotherapy as the only forms of treatment. Others recommend speech therapy before analysis; still others, after it. All agree that psychological factors play a role in speech therapy whether the therapist is aware of it or not. Although some disinclincation or incapacity fully to identify and emphathize with stutterers exists among some analysts, equivalent to the laymen's embarrassment and also equivalent to similar reactions toward the so-called borderline and psychotic disorders, most of the confusion may be attributed to lack of clarity about the essence of the disorder. When that challenge is met in the realm of theory we shall be able to meet the challenge in the realm of practice—an effective therapy. Such therapy will not in all, or even most, cases need to be classical psychoanalysis—it could be analytic psychotherapy. We may vary and improvise the forms of treatment, but the underlying dynamics are not variable.

Chapter 5

Treatment Considerations

In view of what has been said about the psychopathology of stuttering, it may be inferred that the prognosis presents a number of difficult problems. The symptom itself is frequently eliminated, in contrast to other types of conversion symptoms, particularly when the ego is highly differentiated. Often the removal of the symptom itself, and of the unpleasant restrictions resulting from it, is an important aid to the analytic therapy. (Interestingly, the stutter itself, except in the worst cases, is not an important hindrance in treatment, as it frequently improves during therapy.) But of course the greatest difficulty in pscyhoanalytic therapy, long after the removal of the symptom, is the character structure, compounded as it is of compulsive, narcissistic, and oral features. The symptom can be removed; often little more than that can be achieved, occasionally a great deal more. It must be pointed out, however, that while the removal of such a crippling symptom is no small attainment for the therapist, to the patient it is an attainment of immeasurable value.

Such types of treatment as hypnosis, vocal and rhythmic exercises, and various devices of distraction are lacking in pscycho- logical rationale, and I therefore do not regard them as therapies of choice. In speech therapy, which focuses attention exclusively on the symptom, speech is overemphasized; the patient lives, as it were, to speak. Moreover, the symptom, already isolated due to strong resistance, is singled out additionally. This only strengthens its isolation and resistance to treatment. When an improvement or cure of the stutter does occur, it is due to the therapeutic relationship and is not the result of a particular exercise or regimen.

Therapy may take the form of psychoanalysis, analytically

oriented psychotherapy, and psychiatric plus casework therapy conducted by a therapeutic team. The basic principles of psycho-analytic therapy serve as the foundation for the treatment of the character disorders. Special approaches and emphases that are useful and appropriate to the specific needs of the stutterer are integrated with it. One basic modification in analytic therapy for stutterers consists in an active preliminary phase wherein the analyst gives to the stutterer, and what he gives, among other things, is words—something much overvalued by the stutterer. This means talking, and the best content is such safe material as paraphrasing the patient's own productions, sharpening their focus somewhat.

Treatment of the stutterer is aimed at a transformation of his ego organization so that its image and functioning, which were modeled after an organ, may become the image and the functioning of a total organism. The stutterer's inhibitions, symptoms, and character traits have flowed from traumatic experiences; of these the first and most fateful was the nursing and early feeding situation.

First and foremost, the passivity-activity equilibrium has to be repeatedly exposed. For a number of reasons, this is difficult. In accordance with his character, the patient prefers to swallow isolated interpretations and regard them as final answers, rather than synthesize what he is told into usable tools for further observation, validation, and action. For a long time, therefore, what he is told is not very usable to him. His passivity also interfers with comprehension and the application of insight, and contributes to blocking the expression of affect which is crucial for acquisition of insight. Furthermore, expressions of passivity seldom appear directly. They have to be worked out through their defenses, maintained by deep pleasure premiums.

Treatment of the stutterer must be geared to an understanding of the disorder. Merely to give support and to allow expression of aggression are not sufficient. One of the frequently mentioned problems encountered by the therapist is that the stuttering makes him/her uncomfortable and even anxious. These feelings are in part an unconscious reaction to the hostility embedded in the symptom; the understanding of this and especially a concept and a treatment plan geared to it, would make a larger part of the reaction conscious and convert the therapist's fear of the unknown into a greater security with a known condition and a specific plan for its handling. The failure to understand the disorder can produce in the therapist a condition reminiscent of the plight of the medical student who has mastered the techniques of doing a physical examination and taking a history but has as yet not become familiar with any of the syndromes of the various diseases. He has an impulse to ask an infinite number of questions, the answers to each of which have equal value to him; or to do an infinite number of tests. This approach is both needless and nontherapeutic. The general plan of treatment likewise has similar serious pitfalls. The expectation that with unearthing and discovering there will come simultaneous relief of symptoms is altogether futile in this type of disorder, particularly in children. Even classical analysis has to be materially modified in this type of disorder. Insofar as extracting information is a repetition of the familiar battleground with an emasculating mother, it is of primary importance to obtain information but not to extract it.

What follows is a description of a team approach for the clinical treatment of stuttering children. In our clinic work a team of two therapists was assigned to each case. The therapists were analysts, psychiatrists, and/or psychiatric caseworkers. Psychologists were utilized in the initial diagnostic survey. Like the psychiatrists, the caseworkers had been psychoanalyzed and had had advanced experience in casework. All therapists were regularly supervised by the writer.

The decision to have separate therapists for mother and child from the start was based entirely on the assumption of the mother's sense of oneness with her child. Experience has proved further that she was able to relinquish her child if she received a substitute for it, in treatment in the form of her own therapist. This was especially true when the child (a boy in 80 percent of the cases) was assigned to a male therapist. Conversely, when he was given a female therapist the mother frequently interrupted the treatment. We learned further that the mother did very well with a woman therapist, because she was thereby offered a substitutive experience and a basis for a better identification to counteract her own identification with a narcissistic and masochistic woman—her own mother. The girl stutterer did about equally well with either male or female therapist, though here also the mother's attitude was significant. However, it was imperative that the therapist of the mother have the conviction that the mother is a neurotic individual who has a legitimate and often urgent therapeutic need in her own right. Some therapists, possessing great ability for working with children and for identifying with them, were unable to reach these mothers because they lacked such conviction and could not empathize with them.

The initial diagnostic survey began with separate and joint interviews of the child, mother, and father, totaling at least four or five hours. Projective psychological tests were given at first to mother and child; later the father was included. The main objective for obtaining the anamnestic and observational facts was to aid in choosing the most suitable treatment plan in each instance. Determining factors included severity of the neurosis, degree of flexibility and treatability of each patient, motivation, and practical elements. The following treatment plans were employed.

1. *Analysis or psychotherapy of the mother as the only therapy.* Surprisingly, experience proved that this method was efficient for the removal of the stutter as well as for very important characterological changes in the children without direct treatment of them. It was particularly efficient for the younger children but also gave positive results in some adolescents.

2. *Analysis or psychotherapy of the mother and simultaneous psychotherapy of the child.* The children in this category ranged from ages 4 to 15.

3. *Analysis or psychotherapy of the mother and concurrent analysis or psychotherapy of the child.* Children in this series ranged in age from middle through late adolescence. Even in this group it was found that the therapy of the mother facilitated and shortened the course of treatment of the child.

In the beginning of this experience the fathers were not treated formally but were called in occasionally by the therapist of the child in relation to special problems, especially when his behavior was grossly injurious to the child or to the therapy.

The mother frequently came with considerable insight about certain aspects of her relationship to the stuttering child. Other mothers were able to verbalize for the first time during the diagnostic survey their recognition of the causal relation between the child's stutter and the family constellation, especially the mother-child relation. Frequently this insight came to her as a shock and surprise. Her unawareness that the stutterer was felt to be a part of her was the result both of her repressions and of her acting out. Some mothers accepted submissively the suggestion that they be treated; up to that point they had masochistically resigned themselves to their "destiny." Others, on the other hand, were quite enthusiastic that they were about to get treatment for which they were intuitively looking forward. As the treatment of the mother was mandatory, the contact was terminated at the conclusion of the survey whenever she refused to be involved in the therapy. A few exceptions were made when the children were in middle or late adolescence.

The first task in the therapy of the mother was to work through her acceptance of her mixed feelings about her own need for treatment, a need that became more apparent in the discussions of her relationship to her own mother. Next in importance was the exposing and working through of her pent-up anger and anxiety connected with unresolved deep disappointments and frustrations at the hands of her mother. She became aware of these emotions in discussions regarding her separation from her mother and also from her stuttering child. Her fear of separation was frequently convered up by her masochistic submission. Much time and energy had to be spent to uncover these emotions and mental structures. This effort was preliminary to attempts in the development of a realistic sense of self and the formation of new identifications. Her own relationship to her mother was a uniquely important emotional tie, even though this principle is a truism in the most varied disorders. The presence of these strong ties was very subtly disguised because usually the control exerted was quite subtle. These ties and the fears of separation were also related to the patient's rejection of the feminine role, the envy of the male role, and to involvement of the child within the framework of her castration anxiety. She was helped to differentiate between infantile and feminine dependency. One major consequence of this is that she was helped to view her husband not as a disappointing mother image but as a real person to whom she could turn to share in the common problems of rearing their child.

We return now to the problem of bringing the husband, as a real person, into the therapeutic picture. Helping the husband became especially important at the time the mother was ready to work out her relationship with him. The marriage was generally characterized by sado-masochism and frigidity. As a result of the working through of this relationship, a psychological shift frequently took place in it so that the husband was willing to try to relate to the child and the wife in a more positive way. Two approaches were used with the husband-father. At the start of the treatment, when he was in flight as father and husband, he had been deliberately excluded from treatment. Now, to aid him, he was deliberately brought in by the boy's therapist for an occasional interview. With the shifts in the mother's and boy's personalities, positive, constructive qualities in the father were freed for promoting the treatment. He was greatly encouraged as his role was strengthened and he was given the feeling that he was the bulwark of the family, and that he was needed by the therapist to stand by in the treatment of the boy. The several interviews by the boy's therapist exploited the immediate objectives of giving the father information and explanations about the boy's behavior and about the changes that would result in his treatment. In a good many instances this approach was sufficient, but in some cases it was necessary to bring in the father for therapy for himself in a more formal way. This was inevitable when the father developed an active resistance to the treatment as a result of changes in his son and wife.

Insofar as the presenting symptom is not attacked directly—as it is not in analytic psychotherapy—the treatment of the stuttering boy or girl is basically no different from the treatment of any neurotic child. Therefore, speech therapy per se could not be integrated with it. However, in view of the special symptomatology and characterological features presented by the stuttering child, certain modifications in the treatment had to be introduced. Because of his marked separation anxiety an informal and completely permissive atmosphere was necessary. The therapist had himself to speak more frequently and freely and to avoid pressing the child to speak. Such permissiveness was also necessary in order to free the child's expression of anger and aggression through play. The effect of such expressions was particularly noteworthy in the lessening of the stutter after the child acted out some biting, chewing, or smearing activities in relation to toys. The stutter reappeared later in the treatment, especially in the process of working out oedipal conflicts. Frequently the child's behavior regressed quite deeply in therapy, and yet he was able to show well-contained behavior at home.

After a couple of months, sometimes after six months, there was much less concern in the family about the stutter. In a number of instances it had disappeared before that time. The parents were frequently irritated by periods of increased aggressiveness or recurrence of enuresis. Interestingly, the smooth progress of the child's treatment was often an indication that the mother's treatment was progressing smoothly. It was also noted that her regressive behavior in treatment preceded the child's regression, and, further, that by this time the mother was generally aware that she precipitated the regression in the child.

There was considerable acting out by mother and child during treatment. This was due to their basic symbiosis and because of similarities in their attitude about speech as action. The child was thus made to "speak" or act for the mother, and when he was separated by his therapy the mother acted out herself—toward her husband and toward the therapist. In this way her relationships were observed to shift during treatment. Occasionally the mother's negative reactions constituted a threat to the therapy, but it was generally not unsurmountable.

One reason the mother of the stutterer is placed in the center of the therapeutic pattern is that in seeking help for her child she was really seeking it for herself. Usually this was her first indirect application for help for herself, since by that time she had had to endure two severe reactivations of her early separation anxieties: her marriage and the birth of her child. The separation of the mother and son from the state of unconscious fusion freed him and promoted a growth of his ego. The fundamental psychological shift in the family constellation is the result of a loosening of the mother's ties to narcissistic love objects and a turn toward real love objects. In this the working through of her separation anxiety was crucial. Inasmuch as this is a basic complex in the disorder, the mother had to be "seduced" into therapy for herself, although she came seeking it for her child. This indirect treatment of the child is frequently more efficacious than direct therapy because it deals squarely with the basic pathogenesis. An important tool in the therapy of the mother is the interpretation and the working through of transference phenomena. On the other hand, the analysis of complex symptoms and dream interpretations was avoided in the team approach.

The therapeutic team does not aim to cure stuttering per se. The aim rather is to normalize the psychological constellation of the family—the family climate—so as to free each member for further ego maturation. In these circumstances, the stutter ceases to be a family phobia. It loses the excessive charge of anxiety with which it is invested by each member of the family. It may then disappear altogether, or if the stutter reappears it is regarded as an index of some passing emotional disturbance and its intensity is thereby diminished. The family then reacts to it as lightly as to the iterations that appear in the speech of many nonstutterers.

It is possible to apply the psychoanalytic principles and insights to treatment of patients in a group. One such group consisted of adult stutterers. It was revealed that the predominant basis in each patient of this group for seeking treatment was a need to solve some problems connected with being, and the wish to become, a father. Although this was true of this group, obviously this fact cannot be generalized. But a significant aspect of stuttering is thereby demonstrable. It is meaningful only as a reflection of an underlying mental conflict or disequilibrium. When the latter threatens to emerge in consciousness, the stutter worsens and/or becomes a major concern. When the threat is removed either by resolution in consciousness or by the opposite—a deeper re-repression—the stutter either lessens in intensity, disappears, or ceases to be a matter of anxious concern. On the other hand, when the patient is not ready or cannot in a foreseeable future face the conflict, he is not prepared to give up the symptom. Despite his complaints about it he needs it as a shield to protect him against something much more unpalatable or threatening. Hence not all adult stutterers are *ipso facto* to be referred for therapy or are, indeed, treatable. Therefore, for a large number of adult stutterers who cannot have analysis for a variety of reasons, a group method such as this—in contrast to those group methods which attack the symptom directly but vainly—offers considerable though less basic help in a relatively short period of time.

In working with the group therapy of children who stutter, the group approach was employed as adjunctive to individual therapy. The usefulness of the group therapy included an opportunity for a fuller expression of transference reactions, and a possibility for working through the speech phobia and the multiple meanings of the speech symptom. The group was helpful through ego bolstering as a result of identification and experience within the special milieu.

In summary, therapy is based upon insight derived from psychoanalytic investigation of stutterers and of the backgrounds from which they come. The preferred treatment for adult stutterers is individual therapy, analysis or analytic psychotherapy. The treatment goal in relation to the stuttering child is the modification of pathologic character traits by individual therapy—analysis—or analytic psychotherapy of the mother, as the center of the pathogenic constellation of the family of the stutterer, or concurrent individual therapy of the mother and child. The father is involved whenever necessary to the furthering of the treatment.

Chapter 6

Projective Tests in the Treatment of Functional Speech Disorder*

More than ten years ago I was asked by the Child Guidance Clinic of the Jewish Board of Guardians to help them in their Speech Service where they were finding they could not keep patients in treatment for any length of time. The resulting therapeutic project established there was based on insights gained from the psychoanalytic treatment of adolescent and adult stutterers and mothers of stutterers. While the basic therapy was carried out by psychiatric caseworkers under my supervision, I initiated treatment by means of a diagnostic survey, during which I had a number of interviews with the child and both father and mother. This was followed by projective tests of each child.

In the Speech Service in my office I have made these tests mandatory for each child and mother. A few fathers have been tested. There is no question that for purposes of research it would be advisable to test all fathers as well. However, I have had a reluctance to test all fathers routinely. They, like the mothers receive fairly comprehensive anamnestic and psychiatric interviews. I regard these functional speech problems as expressions of total family imbalance. Hence, the treatment aims at a total family reconstellation. While the father contributes to the syndrome both in its causation and maintenance, I nevertheless regard his contribution as quite secondary to that of the mother. Experience has

---

*Originally published in somewhat different form in the *Journal of the Hillside Hospital*, 1954, 3:147–153, under the title "Projective Tests in a Private Service for the Treatment of Functional Speech Disorders."

borne out a conviction acquired very early that the mother must be regarded as the key person in the therapy. She must be treated always either preceding the child or conjointly, or else as the only one, especially if the child is of preschool age. For one thing, it is not practical or feasible to treat all members of a household simultaneously. Since the pathology within the home displaces the father from his logical and traditional place, deliberately not treating him, or what amounts to treating him indirectly through helping the mother resume or find her own natural place within the family, or leaning on him as the mainstay in the family, we have found empirically a sound practice. It is not good for such a family to have all its members look to the therapist as their father for a number of reasons: one of them is that it intensifies the fantasy that they are all siblings.

As will be gathered from what has been said already, the study and treatment of these cases highlight the psychological familial constellation. We might say roughly that the psychopathology within the family is in essence a scrambling of roles within a framework of ideal-object and part-object identifications. The usual classical nosological entities, such as hysterical and obsessional phenomena, are often found in these patients, but they are not the significant dynamic elements. What is both significant and dynamic here are problems of narcissism, orality, masochism, and especially disturbances in identification as the result of or the expression of insufficient ego differentiation. These, then, are what are usually called the borderline or narcissistic states, or perhaps best characterized as "ego-defect neuroses."

With sufficient concentration upon and experience with one broad type of disorder it is possible to have a somewhat focused approach toward both diagnosis and therapy and similarly also toward the use and place of projective techniques. Therapy is fostered from the first contact. We do not approach each new case as a *tabula rasa*. We do not say, "Now, Johnny, let's sit down and find out why you stutter." That's the last thing Johnny wants to do, or for that matter, the last thing his bigger brother and his mother want to do. They want to be given the feeling from the very start that we, the therapists, know all about why he stutters, know it very clearly and well, and that we are there to help him. This attitude is not in contradiction to the Freudian position that to treat is to investigate. As Freud investigated and treated, he always did so with reference to a working hypothesis. To float in the unconscious without a frame of reference is not within the spirit of Freud, but is rather a perversion of it.

What then do I mean by a diagnostic survey, and what are the implications for that very necessary part of it—the projective techniques? The formal diagnosis can generally be made at an early phase; the family constellation can also be sketched out early. The primary aim of the survey is therefore to appraise a number of significant and practical elements. To mention a few: the elements of treatability, the particular constellation and order of treatment and its depth, the suitability of the therapist and the sex of the therapist for the child and the mother; which one of the two patients, for example, shall get the more intensive treatment; the possibility of shifting from one therapist to another and when; and many other practical questions. These are the questions the projective tests aid me in answering. The best results are not obtained by doing "blind" Rorschachs. The experienced psychologist should be taken into the psychiatrist's confidence by being given a sketch of the general background and, in addition, all the necessary questions about special areas wherever possible.

Increasingly, diagnosis has in general been shifting from formal nosological classification which is becoming less meaningful to more specific dynamic factors. Some of these include, for example, the wide field of narcissism and its qualitative characteristics, whether healthy or unhealthy, whether it is satisfied or unsatisfied narcissism. In other words, we want help with problems such as the assaying of the fundamental conflict between narcissistic and external objects—which has the greater investment of libido and aggression. We also need to know the manner in which the aggressive drives function in the psychic economy. How readily do they fuse with libidinal drives, or do they function mainly in isolation? How easily can that energy be deaggressivized or changed into constructive energy? To what objects or their mental representatives do they display their greatest adhesiveness? These questions are practical and of crucial importance in relation to the outcome of therapy, because they underlie such fundamental phenomena as basic trust, and the patient's fixation to traumatic and frustrating events. I am speaking, of course, of the masochism which in treatment leads to the inability to accept help and is the kernel of the negative therapeutic reaction. The answers to these questions determine the particular therapeutic formula that is most suitable to the particular family constellation.

Why do we prefer to get important leads from projective tests? The economy of them was already suggested. The psychologist in one session can probe at different points and come up with samplings of complexes in the depth of the personality in a most remarkable and penetrating manner. Incidentally, the psychologist seems less proficient in appraising the defenses and especially the compensatory and the nonconflictual areas in the personality than in the basic pathology. The former is rapidly assuming more importance in psychiatric evaluations, and it is to be hoped that the projective tests will follow suit and similarly emerge from the traditional exclusive preoccupation with psychopathology. In the second place, an investigative procedure geared to diagnosis is of necessity a more aggressive technique and is experienced as an attack by the patient much more so than investigation which is geared to therapy. In that context, the id is most generally studied within and through the protective layer of defenses. The pace of breaking through these is almost entirely in the hands of the patient. It is difficult to fuse the two approaches by the same professional worker, and it is therefore better to separate them. If the testing psychologist frightens the patient by the Rorschach, as not infrequently happens, especially with the borderline schizophrenic or schizophrenic, he may lose the patient, but the latter may still return to the psychiatrist or analyst. If the latter loses the patient he is not only lost to the therapist but may shun other therapists as well. We have had the experience, especially in the earlier days, with a certain type of neuropsychiatric diagnostic interview which extracted all the information necessary for a diagnoses, leaving the patient limp with fear of any psychotherapy, and in some instances irreparably so. As a matter of fact, in psychiatric interviews with borderline or schizophrenic patients we now even take the anamnesis in very small doses, and not at all in the beginning. It has been my experience when I was studying the family constellation in stuttering that not infrequently after a rich flow of historical data the patient intuitively hit upon an insight, whereupon the flow stopped abruptly.

Speaking of the subject of the danger to the patient from direct probing and into responses from the id, I have had one or two experiences where I could not understand the nature or the depth of the resistance, especially in struggling with the problem of passivity. The Rorschach was able to reveal the underlying schizophrenic process which I could not see clinically. By the same token, as a kind of poetic justice, the Rorschach did not indicate the relatively well-functioning defenses on the surface of the personality.

In addition to the danger to the patient there are also dangers to both the psychologists and psychiatrists. It is quite understandable that such lucid and truly remarkable penetration into the depth of the instinctual life and the unconscious operations of the ego might go to the head of the psychologist, that is to say, to the magical part of it, to inflate his narcissism at the expense of his scientific and human humility. The harm to the psychiatrist is of a different order. He may resort to projective tests too early and too exclusively at the expense of some atrophy to his clinical acumen.

A thorny problem in the daily working life of the psychiatrist and analyst is the problem of semantics. The psychologist is similarly plagued, but has the additional burden of correlating the language of two disciplines. I recall one of the earliest Rorschach reports in my experience. It was written entirely in the pure Rorschach language. Exactly what that is I cannot say, but I felt very much like a student of a foreign language who enjoyed the consciousness of having reached the stage where he could fluently translate at sight. Despite this amusing element I was impressed by the correctness of the findings after a lengthy analysis of the patient. I find those reports most useful which consist mainly of phenomenological descriptions. For example, a statement that the patient is intensely preoccupied with anatomy offers me much more meaning than a statement that the patient is hypochondriacal. The former is more generic, it may serve as a basis for hypochondriasis, but may not be necessarily so, or may have other though related meanings. On the other hand, "hypochondriacal" is more definitive and interpretative, and the interpretation may not be exact. It is also useful to quote some of the patient's replies, especially some that the psychologist cannot interpret. In such a case it is possible that the psychiatrist might find the correct interpretation. For example, a child responded to one of the test cards usually referred to as the "mother" card by saying that he saw a paper weight. Because I supervised the treatment of his mother, I was able to see it as a variation of the dream-screen phenomenon.

Finally, I wish to mention briefly two or three other constructive uses of the report of the projective tests. Gauging progress and the time of termination are self-explanatory, though I have seen some complications. In addition, the psychiatric caseworkers of the team, as well as myself, have found it useful in counteracting the absorption in certain problems at the expense of a blurring of the total picture periodically to reread all the psychological findings. This helped in seeing the clinical picture whole again as well as integrating a particular problem more meaningfully in the total context.

Chapter 7

Clinical Considerations

Diagnosis of a functional symptom is complicated by its relation to the subject's character structure, the habitual ego and superego patterns. By definition, no symptom is possible without some failure of the ego. In the pure neuroses, or psychoneuroses, this weakness is minimal and circumscribed, is not seen directly but only recognized indirectly by the presence of the symptom. But in the character disorders the ego in its specific functional and sensory aspects is itself impaired. The stuttering symptom, then, may reflect either a psychoneurosis or a character disorder. But in the latter case the stutter takes on a different quality—it becomes less a symptom but rather more like a trait. It is then less ego-alien, more acceptable to the ego. Because there is less motivation for its removal, the patient does not complain of it spontaneously. When, under these circumstances, the patient is nevertheless forced to come for help he is quite resistant. He wishes to be told that the symptom is not curable, or else that it does not matter; or, still differently, that he wishes it to be removed in mid-air, so to speak, and that there is nothing at all he has to complain about as regards his personality or his life. In other words, he wishes to be left alone.

Several clinical features are worth noting in the development of stuttering. First, unlike the classical neuroses, the symptoms of which precipitate during adolescence, stuttering emerges either shortly after the onset of speech or when the child begins school. It then continues without interruption through the latency period and beyond. Second, it is frequently and consistently presented by the patient as a monosymptomatic disorder; the stutterer may have many inhibitions besides the symptom, but for the most part they

65

are totally unknown to him. In fact, inhibition invades the speech function itself, for the stutter is in essence an unsuccessful attempt at inhibition. Another common defense takes the form of phobias for speech situations. The inhibitions and phobias are out in the open only as far as speech is concerned, but hidden as far as they affect parallel adjustment in social, sexual, and occupational spheres. The fact that they remain hidden behind one symptom, which alone mobilizes the conscious attention and concern of the patient, accounts in large part for the great intractability of the symptom. Although the above-mentioned traits and symptoms are not confined to the stutterer alone, in him their relative concentration and expression through speech are unique.

The secondary gain through illness—the satisfaction derived from a symptom after it is formed, apart from the deeper satisfaction that caused it to form—was rarely observed in patients who were already in treatment. A stuttering surgeon once remarked to a colleague that his patients, especially women who admired him very much, referred to his stutter as cute. He, it might be noted, was not in treatment. The large majority of patients in treatment were eager to be rid of their disturbing symptom; this same desire can also be attested to by the existence of so many speech clinics.

A stutter is often produced when the speaker is placed at a disadvantage, thus indicating that he acts so in order to gratify his own severe superego. Despite the painfulness of speaking and stuttering, some stutterers can and do secondarily extract a kind of satisfaction in such situations, such as being pitied or getting gratification from keeping the audience tense and waiting. These gains are generally unconscious but may be made conscious. In some cases the pain and humiliation of stuttering will be used to relieve guilt feelings related to other gratifications, or to arouse pity. They can also be utilized more or less consciously as a spiteful aggression against a parent who overvalues the function of speech.

Both the fantasy wishes and the defenses set up against them seek different forms of expression, including speech. In the unconscious of the stutterer the final aim of the magical act of speaking is to attain the fulfillment of the narcissistic ideal. The defenses, on the other hand, attempt to block both the expression of this aim and its magical attainment through speech. The stutter therfore means a partial expression and symbolic attainment of the wish and a partial blocking of both. When either the expression or the blocking is complete, there is no stutter. This happens both in health and in psychosis. In the former it is the result of unambivalent, deliberate choice to speak or be silent, and in the latter is the result of failure in the strength of repression.

A few instances of bizarre stuttering have been seen in disturbed, masochistic, and prepsychotic patients. With the outbreak of the psychosis based on giving up many of the defenses, the stutter ceased altogether. On the other hand, for the same type of patient, although therapy at times intensified the stutter, it nevertheless robbed it of its bizarre nature.

Stuttering is not a constitutional or hereditary disorder. All the eivdence of constitutionality given—rigidity, persistence, very early onset of symptoms such as feeding difficulties, restlessness, overactivity, and behavior indicative of regression to intrauterine life—have been observed in infants during the first half year as reactions to a rejecting environment, often very subtly disguised; and these symptoms have disappeared when the atmosphere in the home and the handling of the child were changed.

Ribble (1941), in prolonged studies of young infants suffering from unsatisfied "stimulus hunger," found two types of reaction. The first type is general negativism: refusal to nurse, anorexia, failure to assimilate food; muscular rigidities and resistance to extension of torso and extremities; and shallow breathing. The second type, the more serious, is the depressive or regressive type. It includes feeble attempts at nursing, followed by stuporous sleep; loss of sucking reflex; pallor; asthenia; regurgitation and diarrhea; and irregular breathing with occasional apnea. After the third month, more discernible affective responses appear—temper outbursts and evidences of anxiety. The resemblence between the clinical picture of "constitution" and that resulting from unsatisfied "stimulus hunger" is striking. I believe that the infantile reactions to inadequate mothering are the precursors of the so-called "constitution" of the stutterer.

Speech pathologists of the eclectic school (Szondi, 1932; Seemann, 1934) emphasize the "constitution" of the stutterer. Although they regard it as hereditary, which I do not, the observations are sound. They mention muscular restlessness, hyperkinesis, hypertensions, and poor coordination in the speech organs and other parts of the body; spastic intestinal symptoms; irregular and shallow respiration; and hypersensitiveness to light and sound stimuli. In many cases there is also a tendency to asthenia, fatigability, excessive need for sleep and food. Neurologically, this syndrome is referred to as amphotonia—i.e., stimulation of both the sympathetic and parasympathetic branches of the automatic nervous system.

A word about the question of cerebral dominance in the etiology of stuttering (Orton, 1928). Although statistical reports vary, there probably is a greater percentage of native left-handedness among stutterers than among nonstutterers. There is also probably a greater confusion about handedness among stutterers who have not been changed than among nonstutterers. Here enters the complicating thought of at least one writer (Parson, 1924), who alleges that eyedness is the primary determinant of handedness. Psychologically there is a connection between the two, but which is primary we are not prepared to say. We can only offer one empiric observation. In the stutterer and in the compulsive character there is much ambivalence (love, hate; good, bad; masculine, feminine). There is also evidence of the unconscious association of masculine with right and feminine with left. It would seem logical to postulate that psychologic ambivalence may be expressed somatically as confusion in handedness, eyedness, etc. May not this problem be primarily one of psychologic rather than neurologic dominance?

The psychoanalysis of stutterers permitted the observation of certain defenses. The most stable and comparatively least painful defense, one observed with great frequency, was of distancing in interpersonal relations. Love objects were unconsciously enjoyed through their mental representations, though actual relationships were superficial and offered a minimum of conscious pleasure.

More baffling was the masochistic defense, which could best be understood in terms of its dynamic content. The wish to become one with the idealized phallic mother was countered by two fears: the fear of complete regression into passivity, as a kind of inertia or death, and its opposite—the fear of getting enough satisfaction to be stimulated or maneuvered sooner or later into activity and, finally, separation. Against these fears the patient would defend himself by unconsciously maintaining a passive attachment to a "traumatizing" mother figure, a distorted version of his actual mother. He became one with her—treated himself aggressively and harshly as he felt she would treat him—and projected this image onto others. An arrangement such as this offered several gratifications. The real mother, even as she was distorted in the child's mind, was authentic. His wished-for ideal mother figure was not authentic since she was part of a dangerous outside world and could not be trusted. Besides, the relationship offered a vent for much pent-up aggression through complaints and accusations, expressed or unexpressed. It was impossible to feel or express oneself in that way toward a nonfrustrating parental figure, at least not without much guilt. Since this defense protected the patient chiefly from separation anxiety, gave him the illusion of activity, and served other needs as mentioned above, it offered him much unconscious satisfaction which overbalanced the consciously felt galling dominations, frustrations, and failures.

The following traits of the stutterer had features of both masochistic and compulsive reactions: pseudoactivity, a kind of busyness to avoid anxiety associated with waiting or with real activity; being busy to ascertain the wished-for incorporation, following which it was hoped endless passivity might be enjoyed under more ideal circumstances, or pseudoaggression; and behavior actually provocative or deemed so, aiming among other goals at caricaturing genuine productive activity in extreme terms and thus laughing it out of court and avoiding it. Related to this pseudoaggression was phallic exhibitionism, the character trait of acting as if one's body were a phallus. These patients like to strut or to appear to be doing something for others. Their real aim, however, was passivity—to be incorporated by and lose themselves in the onlookers.

At bottom the chief characteristics of a personality functioning unconsciously as an organ are inhibitions and passivity. For example, at one point a patient constantly postponed telephoning, ostensibly because he disliked to stutter over the telephone. Actually, his stutter represented a wish to block a call which in turn would necessitate pursuing an active curiosity and then planning a course of action. The stutter thus represented an inhibition in the area of speech which simultaneously fortified the inhibition of the total personality.

Many other activities were modeled after their oral aims and inhibitions. For example, most stuttering patients, feeling discontent with their state of adjustment to reality, made many efforts at self-improvement. Analysis of their activity and of their failure to attain the desired goal revealed some of the fundamental defects of their ego functions. For instance, it is self-evident that to solve a problem it is essential to have a feeling that one has a right to solve it. But when the stutterer's self-image was that of a dependent part of another person, his feeling in the face of such a task was that he was being dangerously presumptive and provocative. He therefore always felt that he was usurping the authority of "headquarters"—that the executant functions of the ego were outside himself. By the same token, these patients felt that they had not the "wherewithal," a term frequently used to denote independent action, mind, voice, sexual adequacy, or total self. The end result was hesitation and blocking of action or behavior. The same held true for the functions of imagination, volition, and creativity. As stated above, however, within the scope of performing an assignment in which the individual functioned as a faithful part of a larger entity, considerably greater plasticity of thinking and action was available to the stutterer.

Apart from having a right to—or its psychic equivalent, having an organ for—independent functioning, it is also essential that one have a clear perception of a problem requiring solution. Such clarity was obscured, in different degrees of intensity, by the startling fact that many stuttering patients acted in real life and in treatment as if they were walking in their sleep, or acting out a dream. The dream began with a wish for complete passivity and was merged with an anxious escape from the destructive consequences of such extreme passivity (libidinal sleep into defensive sleep). This was analogous to the merging of their expectant, "waiting" silence with anxious, fearsome silence. In real life one often noted their wishful thinking and daydreaming, accompanied by inhibition and general ineffectuality. It was as if they were acting out their wish to "sleep away" their lives, a combination of nursing and running away. In treatment, it was common to note amnesia for the content of their therapeutic hours, frequent actual drowsiness, and occasional falling asleep.

In these patients the same difficulties pertained to problems of volition, imagination, or action. Blocking the beginning of words and sentences—the essence of the stutter—tended to recur at every new step in making use of the various ego functions. It seemed as if all activity, mental and motor, had come to bear the imprint of the struggle with oral aggression which first emerged during nursing, even before and independent of the eruption of the teeth—the usual stated period of emergence of oral sadism.

Repeatedly the patient's fundamental conflicts oscillated between efforts to adjust to inner and outer pressures, with an ego image of an organ and efforts to function with an ego image of an organism. On the emotional plane the stuttering patient tried to establish feelings about mental and motor activity as different and distinct from oral destructiveness or passive annihilation. With regard to aims he had to shift from archaic fantasies of passivity to realistic plans of activity; to renounce distorted notions of activity and of passivity. In this way a foundation could be laid for growth. Sooner or later the patient encountered the need to identify with his therapist. Identification is a fundamental mechanism of growth. Once more a significant struggle with his fixation took place. The only technique he "knew" was through becoming one with the therapist by passive submission. Because this wish was felt as nursing or yielding or being consumed and overpowered, even annihilated, he often fell prey to shame or conscience qualms, or even to fears of physical attack, the last representing the well-known homosexual panic.

Incidentally, it was in this context that obscenity of the anal type often emerged. Intrapsychically, obscene words represented reprimands and threats of punishment by the primitive conscience. The early ego state which functioned with the fantasy-wish to be incorporated orally and anally was derisively equated with abdominal contents or feces and finally threatened with expulsion. Externally, obscenity stood for a kind of defense against the same passivity. The stutter, then, encompasses an attempt to block the expression of the wish, the reprimand, and the defense, plus a partial expression of all three.

In 1913, Federn presented to the Vienna Psychoanalytic Society a case of bronchial asthma, which Freud discussed. According to Rank's report, Freud thought that Federn's case should not be classed with hysteria; he suggested calling such cases "fixation hysterias." The Minutes of the Society (Nunberg and Federn, 1975, p. 146) report Freud as saying, "Cases like this have particular predisposing conditions. These organ neuroses tack themselves onto hysteria, to be sure, but they have to be separated from it. Erotogenic stresses on organs overwhelm the psychic mechanism, forcing the neurosis to manifest itself in organic ways. These neuroses differ from the usual hysteria in that they do not represent repression, but, rather, infantilism."

Two questions present themselves here in relation to the stutterer: precisely what is encompassed by the rather large order of infantile fixations; and, what, if any, relations do these fixations bear to other pathologic mechanisms, especially regression, and to symptom formation in the form of conversion? It seems to me that the dominant impulse interfered with by fixation is that of oral incorporation (drinking, chewing, breathing) in both its active and passive aspects. From the structural standpoint, the dominant expression inhibited by fixations is that of ego emergence and evolution from the id or other primordial energy substrata.

From the general psychopathology of the neuroses, it has been established that the point at which instinctual and structural expressions lead the individual to have similar conflicts and experience anxiety, or its somatic equivalents, is one where separation is involved. It begins with physical birth, is re-experienced with eating, weaning, training, locomotion; with the onset of speech, denoting the birth of the ego; and reaches its height at the oedipal period in the form of castration anxiety. The last is a link in a chain of anxieties in which important earlier links are the primal scene and the development of the phallic phase. Both merge with the accentuated oral phase and become "oralized." In my experience, separation anxiety in its varied forms, but especially in the context of the fantasy of the mother-child symbiosis, constitutes what I believe to be the nub of what Freud referred to as "infantilism." Federn, in a personal communication, confirmed this idea. He wrote:

> "I have seen quite a few cases of stuttering; all cases were provoked by some castration anxiety, by masturbation and by fear of telling it to the mother, by the fear that somebody might know it. I remember a case which clearly began after the child watched the intercourse of the parents. It is interesting that the lowest level is the feeding, where the relationship of mouth and breast has the connotation of phallic castration and the higher level is the conflict during the period of articulation, promoting that which is the real castration complex."

Now, as to the second question: Do these infantile fixations stand alone, i.e., emerge in their original form and remain so, or are they—as is the case in the classical neurosis—a point to which later developed instinctual and ego manifestations return and express themselves anew in a reorganized and distorted fashion under the primacy of the earlier organization? Here, differences of opinion exist.

In my own experience, I have observed a wide range of complexity in the defensive process against the oral and the other instinctual impulses seeking expression in the stutter. Hardly ever have I noticed in the stuttering act the blissful faces suggestive of the relaxed attitude of the satisfied nursling or of the adult postcoital state, alluded to by Coriat. Even in stutterers who indulged in oral perversions without any guilt, any desire to regress to the level of pure oral erotism or oral sadism was instantly blocked by inhibitions in the speech. It seems to me that a more valid distinction than the degree of impulse as against defense within the stuttering symptom involves rather the nature of each. Specifically, I mean the following: the pregenital disorder discussed here represents disturbances of specific physiological automatisms (of speech, of breathing, or general muscular actions), that is, of ego functions which have evolved from the pre-ego (id, or other sources) state. The arrest, partial development, or deviation in the ego in this process of transformation due to specific environmental, traumatic, or consti-tutional factors I refer to as a fixation, an ego fixation. The stutter is the result of an attempt to defend against this fixation. Thus, when a stutterer wants unconsciously to bite or suck when he is supposed to speak, a conflict ensues, the result of which contains some elements of biting or sucking and also elements of attempts to block or inhibit such expression. But even these fixations do not threaten to return from repression unless they themselves are called in as a defense following regression from an advanced ego and libido position, especially the oedipal phase. The fixations hardly ever threaten by their own weight alone, though that weight may be substantial and should not be underestimated.

The idea of a restitutive motif in narcissistic or ego-defect disorder* helped me to explain a number of otherwise obscure phenomena. For example, the phenomenon of perseveration in stuttering is generally regarded as the primary disorder, the so-called dysphemia of the nonanalytic school, and the tonic and spastic symptoms as reactive or secondary. But I submit that from the standpoint I am now discussing, it seems that genetically and dynamically the perseveration itself is an attempt at correcting or containing a tendency toward diffuseness of thought associations and other aspects of primary-process thinking. Such an explanation might account for the fact that perseveration and diffuseness are often found alongside each other in much the same way that anxiety is found to emerge alongside the symptom that is intended to contain it.

The stutterer's striving to regress from object-related to non-object-related speech represents the flight or withdrawal from objects. This flight is countered by an opposing impulse for closeness. The conflict is reflected in the stuttering symptoms. When constancy is maintained either at close or normal range or at a distance greater than usual (nonobject-related speech), no stuttering occurs. It is my contention that the situation here is identical with what Freud postulated for speech in the schizophrenic, though

---

*Freud mentions the aim of restitution in the symptomatology of schizophrenia in his discussion of the Schreber case (1911b). He elsewhere (1915) refers to schizophrenia as one of a number of narcissistic states. I have explicitly extended the implication of restitution to the narcissistic disorder under discussion and I believe it applies to other, if not all, narcissistic conditions.

in this instance he explicitly connected schizophrenia with other narcissistic disorders (1915).

Thus in the unconscious psychic life of both there is a corresponding libidinal improverishment of the object representation, but paradoxically in the preconscious where the verbal ideas correspond to the object, these verbal ideas or words are hypercathected. This brings to mind Ferenczi's remark (1911) that obscene words retain a hallucinatory quality in that they compel the hearer to imagine the object they denote. The stutterer, in a sense, also contents himself with words in place of things and people. The urge to regression, which causes the struggle and the stutter, serves a restitutive purpose—namely, to check the flight and regain closeness to the object, psychic as well as real. In other words, the stutterer maintains his contact with reality—i.e., the object in speaking situations—through the stutter. Hospitalized psychotics who have broken down from reality and who have been stutterers up to that time of breakdown hardly ever stutter.

Stutterers are very frequently the compulsive type in their personality structure. Freud (1913) called attention to the connection between the compulsion neurosis and the precocious development of the ego in relation to that of the libido. It appears probable that this precocity is due to traumata either at the oral level or which culminate at the oral level, as in the case of the stutterer. The early awakening of the ego is also, I believe, a restitutive phenomenon. Because of the apparent urgency of the ego's mobilization and the repression of the precipitating events, it is difficult for this early ego to relinquish its hold and mature. It is not, of course, the precocity per se that is important, but the resultant tenacity of the immature ego. Thus, especially, it uses an excess of aggressive energy which it finds difficult to neutralize. It is therefore unsuited for realistic adaptation and can express itself largely on a fantasy plane. This leads to a personality that functions better and preferably in relative isolation.

In summary, psychoanalysis has unearthed a number of fundamental links in the chain of causation in stuttering. Psychoanalysis, dealing with deep phenomena which operate unconsciously, aims at elucidating fundamental meanings of inhibitions and symptoms; it aims also at disclosing the nature of the disorganizing influences and the bases for their maintenance. Manifest phenomenological expressions of this disorder are obviously an indispensable part of our knowledge of it; they have a further usefulness for checking the validity of our concepts from the depth and for stimulating us to make the latter more comprehensible and comprehensive. But standing isolated from their roots, manifest phenomena offer us very little indeed for understanding, for treatment, and for prevention. They cannot substitute for the knowledge of unconscious motivations and for unconscious mental processes. Neither can the realm of the unconscious mental life be skipped over, overlooked, or denied in other ways. One can do that only at the peril of sterility in comprehending phenomena of human behavior in general and of psychosomatic disorders in particular.

Part II

Other Selected Papers

Chapter 8

Observations on a Primary Form of Anhedonia*

Anhedonia

Definition: *The lack of, or the inability to have, conscious pleasure.*

Example: *An individual who at a social gathering behaves in an aloof manner and who, in his feelings, is unaware of any pleasure. However, upon his return home, he can mentally re-experience some of the events with considerable pleasurable accompaniment.*

Related concepts: *This state is the usual affective component of the schizoid state. It is related to, but has to be distinguished from, depression, apathy, and anxiety.*

A specific form of anhedonia appears clinically as a chronic state of lack of conscious pleasure—distinct from psychological states having a quality of painfulness—often punctuated by acute anxiety, unconsciously utilized to re-establish the chronic state whenever its maintenance is threatened by pleasure or by depression. Nosologically, the patients in whom this state has been observed were all schizoid personalities. Their symptomatology prominently included stuttering, homosexual perversions, gastrointestinal disorders (pep-

*Originally published in the *Psychoanalytic Quarterly*, 1949, 18:67–78.

tic ulcer, intestinal spasm, jaundice, diarrhea), and migraine. These symptoms are not considered pathognomonic. Dynamically, this state of inhibited fulfillment stems from those manifestations of orality that derive from narcissistic fixations of libido and its two main forms of expression—identification and projection—in contradistinction to oral regression from object libido. Objectively, the manifestations of this emotional state are described by many terms: withdrawal, detachment, isolation, alienation, chronic aloofness, listlessness, emotional block, etc. A term adequately descriptive of the subjective state is lacking.

Anhedonia (*an* = not, *hedone* = pleasure), an absence of pleasure, was first used by the French psychologist Theophile Ribot (1897) in contradistinction to analgesia, or absence of pain. As Ribot defined it, it is "an insensibility relating to pleasure alone." It seemed to me an apt term to adopt because of the negative quality in the patients' descriptions of their subjective states. The qualification "primary" was added to delimit the type of patients: schizoid characters who, because of very early fixations, felt a sense of distance and a lack of pleasure in all their relationships. Anhedonia may be a chronic state or experienced transiently as a strong reaction to a painful frustration; in both cases there is indifference to objects, absence of closeness, and a feeling of emptiness. These problems do not include inhibited fulfillment based upon oedipal guilt, moral masochism (Freud, 1924), which excludes success (Freud, 1916), or so-called neurotic depressions.

Primary anhedonia is a clinical entity. In psychoeconomic terms it is a consequence of failure of libidinal investment within the conscious ego boundaries due to instinct defusion and the resultant fixation of libido to an unconscious, primitive ego. This ego—the narcissistic ideal ego (Freud, 1914)—is undifferentiated from the magical, omnipotent mother image. This fixation, in turn, is a reaction to specific intolerable environmental conditions during the earliest phases of the child's life. According to Federn (1952; see also Bergmann, 1963), the psyche is rendered unable to withstand the injurious effects of the claims of libido because of traumatic experiences; hence, libido is withdrawn from the boundary of ego cathexis.

Anhedonia can be differentiated from other affective states on the same ego-libido level (anxiety, apathy, depression). Anhedonia may, under certain circumstances, be transformed into any one of these.

Anxiety is that painful state associated with the imminent breaking away of the libido from secure narcissistic images and flowing in the direction of real objects regarded with doubt and fear. What is feared is the danger of ego impoverishment or annihilation. These are the crises or panic reactions which occur in the course of the anhedonic state when either patient or object makes a conscious effort to establish a close and steady relationship. The patient is attempting unconsciously to shift the cathexis from the narcissistic ideal of the ego to a real object, resulting in an awareness of separation, expressed in feelings of emptiness. Since real objects are regarded as destructively aggressive (a projection of the subject's oral aggression), an attempted object relationship results in a panicky fear of destruction. A classic example of this phenomenon is the homosexual panic in latent homosexual patients.

Apathy is the subjective state denoting absence of both painful and pleasurable feelings; it represents a still further degree of libido introversion. The anhedonic patient, although not enjoying positive pleasure from objects, derives some tangible though inarticulate satisfactions from unconscious narcissistic libido fixations and from the operation of ego defenses, including a sense of reality, despite some degree of paranoid coloring in the personality.

The distinction between anhedonia and depression is more difficult to make. Depression may be described as an affective state in which the libido is withdrawn from objects and replaced by aggression; thus identification is equivalent to destruction through incorporation. In anhedonia, while the relationship is also one of destructive identification, it is to *representations* of objects, the libido remaining narcissistically bound. This constitutes the defensive distance of anhedonia and is the chief difference between depression and anhedonia. The absence of the defensive distance permits love objects of the depressive character to have a relatively greater degree of reality, resulting in ambivalence of feeling and behavior. The anhedonic feeling of hollowness results from the defensive distance from real objects and the unconscious ego. Once the gap is lessened, a part of the defensive aggression emerges from repression; a certain quantity is projected, the paranoid trends constituting a secondary defense. If both defenses fail, depression follows. When depression and anhedonia are mixed in various proportions in the same subject, the defensive function of the latter has failed in part. The depressive is more active in his pursit of objects. Both have traumatic fixations compulsively repeated; however, the traumata and their consequences differ. In anhedonia the trauma relates to the earliest (preverbal) relationship to the mother. In depression, such an early trauma is frequent, but in addition there is frustration in the relationship with the father during the oedipal period. Ego functions relating to reality testing and object libido have both reached more advanced stages in the depressive. Crises in object relations are expressed by the anhedonic patient in the form of anxiety or panic reactions; by the depressive patient in depression or in elation followed by depression.

Some Physical and Mental Manifestations of the Anhedonic State

The anhedonic patient typically looks and acts younger than his age, often has a superficial, ingratiating charm, occasionally with animation. Restlessness and clumsiness are frequently observed in patients who nevertheless have a good sense of rhythm. Self-consciousness and exhibitionism are common, sometimes with studied appearance and attitudes, and fixed facial expressions. Speech is rapid, poorly articulated, sometimes suggesting baby talk. The content is often empty, circumstantial chatter, delivered in the flat or monotonous tone of a soliloquy. The men are withdrawn, the women more unrestrainedly emotional, less reticent. Usually the trend is of whining querulousness; more rarely of superior or tacitly reproachful martyrdom. Their self-esteem oscillates between feelings of worthlessness and overestimation, between masochistic submission and omnipotence. They dream of being abused, slighted, or unjustly treated.

Varying quantities of libido are fixated to introjected, idealized, narcissistically invested images, to which objects chosen in reality correspond. The more real relationships become, the more frustrating they are. Individuals are valued only as long as they fit into a realistically unattainable, idealistic frame of reference. To avoid painful disillusionment these patients gradually renounce objects and pleasurable experiences. In transference, this renunciation is a resistance which is expressed in poverty of thoughts, silence, apathy, insatiable demands for love, explosive hostility, distrust, and flight from therapy.

The crises are symptomatically expressed in somatic conversions (abdominal cramps, nausea, diarrhea, headaches), or in action (usually verbal aggression or flight), the latter generally based upon unconscious provocations for making the object appear as the frustrater (Bergler, 1945).

An interesting sequence was the appearance of headaches during the ambivalent struggle resulting from closeness to the love object. As illusions about the real object are resolved, the possiblity of projecting narcissistic images on it is lessened, and the unconscious mental ego reinvested with libido. Headache is concomitant with the repression of aggression toward the real object during the struggle. The unconscious fight represents the ambivalent incorporation and destruction of the object and the acting out of the destructive process, through identification, until the object representation is expelled. The expulsion takes the form of diarrhea or vomiting, discharging the incorporated object and relieving the sense of guilt. These observations agree with Nunberg's (1926), that symptoms referable to the heart and lungs are substitutes for alimentary processes, the specific organ system for localization of oral-anal fantasies. In headaches the organic unit of aggression is also muscle spasm, but it involves the muscles of the cerebral blood vessels.

When the anhedonic defense fails and aggression emerges openly, such explosions are succeeded by anxiety, followed by emptiness and lifelessness. The struggle against such eruptions is evidenced chronically in muscular tonicity (Reich, 1933) or, acutely, in storms of purposeless muscular activity. In a few instances the reactions resembled grand mal, petit mal, or epileptic equivalents.

The headaches resemble the syndrome of migraine, suggesting the possiblity that similar psychopathology may underlie at least some cases of migraine. When cathexis upon a real object exceeds the patient's usual capacity, and headaches and psychomotor explosions do not suffice to discharge the liberated libido and diffuse aggression, anxiety persists or is partly expressed in cardiac symtomatology, partly by fear of death. When all these fail, depression sets in. Except for crises, there is no anxiety; the inward deviation of libido is ego-syntonic, hence without painful affect— only absence of pleasure. Anxiety is the indicator of instability in the anhedonic state.

Clinical Material

A man of 30 was referred for analysis because he had stuttered since early childhood. Every important adaptation he had to make had to be postponed until treatment had overcome his stuttering. He had had a number of love affairs with divorcees of the "extrovert type," usually older than himself, because they initiated and carried the greater share of the conversation. He pursued them intensively, established a sexual relationship, and quickly lost interest.

He was quite aloof and detached, a man of few words expressed in a jumbled manner and rapid pace, with a clonic and tonic stutter. He appeared calm, but inwardly he was tense and impatient. He reacted to painful situations by repressing feelings and by postponing action, by running out or staying away. His life was devoid of any real, sustained, pleasurable relationship with anyone. When lonely he occasionally visited a bar, and socially a cocktail was indispensable to lessen his tension and restlessness. This chronic state was occasionally altered by excitement in anticipation of a relationship with a woman, and by painful affects when it terminated.

The patient's parents were divorced when he was three years old. He remained with his mother; his brother, three years older, was taken by the father. The mother, seemingly infantile, and unable to cope with the care of a boy of five, gave him up for adoption. The patient never saw her afterwards and he lived alone with his foster mother, whom he described as a "controlling" and "scheming" woman. The foster father was psychopathic. The patient traveled with his foster parents, and he attended many schools in the United States and Europe. The foster parents were divorced when he was about 10 years old.

He recalled vividly two events from his early childhood: being beaten by his grandmother and expressing a wish to be dressed like a girl. This transvestite wish recurred in his later life, increasing in complexity as he grew older, often serving as a fantasy to stimulate masturbation and induce sleep. In adult life he derived the greatest pleasure from the fantasy of applying lipstick with a brush. Asked what the brush was composed of, he answered angrily: "I suppose you will call me a cocksucker." The transvestite fantasy was analyzed as his identification with his own frustrating mother. He portrayed her also as being frustrated by men: being left and not given the love and money she desired. This fantasy served the multiple purpose of providing direct libidinal gratification, aggression toward real objects, narcissistic gratification, and masochistic submission, humiliation, and guilt.

His deepest wishes, expressed in fantasies, revealed the narcissistic regression which always followed his attempts to form object-libidinal relationships. He fantasied himself as the hero of a novel in which a miner working deep in a mine is the sole fertile male survivor following an atomic bomb explosion. That the magical omnipotence and phallic exhibitionism are equated both with fecundity and with the ever-flowing breast of the ideal mother was suggested by another fantasy in which he landed by airplane on an island in the Pacific after all of its inhabitants had been killed by a bomb. He was wearing his most attractive feminine garments, but there was no one to see him.

In analysis he was frequently silent initially, waiting to be "given a start" (oral dependence). Failing this, the expectant silence became a struggle to suppress aggressive thoughts and words resulting from disappointment (inhibited oral aggression). He would complain frequently of hunger and fatigue, both of which would disappear by the end of the hour. On these occasions he would speak of feeling dirty (coprophagia). On the day following the analysis of the fantasy about lipstick, the patient telephoned he was ill. When he returned the next day he announced that during the evening following the last hour, while in the company of a woman friend, he was suddenly seized with cramps and had a diarrhea, continuing the following day, which he attributed to "ptomaine." This symptom represented the elimination of the dangerous introjected love object in the transference. Uncomfortable in the analytic hour, he sought a woman to escape and, he said, to "show up" the analyst. The diarrhea and flight (reactions to passive dependent wishes) also represented an aggressive defense against an infantile object regarded as hostile and destructive, which could not be assimilated and had to be disposed of as quickly as possible.

What this patient felt was absence of real pleasure rather than pain. What he recalled of his early life, and related without feeling, was the experience of leaving and being left. He could therefore not risk any new attachments and the danger of being abandoned again. Noteworthy is the fixation upon oral deprivation and its perpetuation through the repetition compulsion (Freud, 1920a), which seems to have the purpose of actively overcoming a hurt reacted to passively; by actively depriving others, he felt himself in the role of the magically omnipotent mother.

An attractive, single woman of 31, appearing much younger than her age, sought treatment for a gradual intensification of anxiety. Following separation from her lover, phobias left her unable to work and disturbed her sleep. She had difficulty in eating and was unable to remain alone. The patient had had similar episodes in her love life and in her relationship with superiors at work.

This patient's mother was a self-centered, vain, impulsive woman in her late forties when the patient, the youngest of six children, was born. About the same time the patient's older sisters were having their own children. The family scene reminded the patient of living in a hotel. There was much buzzing life all about her while she always had a feeling of loneliness. The father, weaker than the mother in making decisions, was overburdened with eking out a living. The paternal grandmother, the most consistently loving person in the family, was old and sickly when the patient was born. The patient was the toy of her mother and the older children, who babied her but neglected her needs. In addition to the fundamental trauma, which was the lack of consistent, loving care oriented to the child's need, this patient in infancy had repeated experiences of witnessing the sexual activities of the older siblings, one of whom was psychopathic.

Soon after beginning treatment, a series of painful experiences occurred, all following the same pattern. She would attract a man and start an affair shortly after meeting him. Soon she would develop a strong urge to get the man to make a decision about marriage, and would then complain that he broke off the relationship. Each time she would suffer anxiety, insomnia, and an inability to work or remain alone. For a time marriage became the *sine qua non* of the worthwhileness of life, and then sole criterion of a successful analysis. In her approach to men there was a directness and a lack of the usual sense of modesty. She had a predilection for fellatio, and in intercourse she was frigid. The first time she attained an orgasm she made involuntary chewing motions with her mouth.

It was necessary for her to continue working for financial and therapeutic reasons. She was frequently involved in a struggle with her superior who, she complained, was not giving her enough recognition, and babied her, yet gave her more work than the others. When an announcement was made that her superior would soon leave the service, she reacted with an attack of anxiety for which she was taken for treatment to the infirmary of the place where she worked. From there she fled in anxiety to the room in which she lived, and where at other times she was unable to remain alone. This attack occurred at a moment when she had a burst of warm feeling for her superior. During the following hour she expressed a growing conviction that she could not tolerate permanence in a relationship. She recalled how content she had been for several years as an impermanent clerk at a low salary. As soon as she was appointed a civil servant in a permanent category, she instigated a quarrel, which at the time seemed quite justified, and nearly resigned. Perhaps it was also the permanency of marriage she could not accept. As she was leaving, she experienced a sensation in her abdomen as if something were being torn out of her; she recalled her feeling of anger, as a small child, whenever she was given enemas, which she resented as a forcible removal of abdominal contents.

Her "spells" or "crises" had a trancelike quality during which she had been observed closing the door, putting out the light and smoking, hunched up in one corner of the settee. This, like her impulsive running to her room from work, may be regarded as fulfilling her need for restoration of the status quo through a reincorporation or rebirth. This trancelike state came at a time when the existence of the unconscious narcissistic ideal state was threatened with being shattered by a sudden burst of warm feeling for someone. Running away from work acted out the separation from or expulsion of the threatening love object, and returning to her room acted out the reinvestment of the narcissistic ideal.

During such a crisis the patient stared into space. She often shook herself as if to rouse herself from an enveloping fantasy. She avoided looking at the analyst. Her speech was thick, like baby talk. She showed changes in skin sensation. One arm might get very cold while the other perspired freely, according to the association with absence or presence of contact. Thus the loss of libido cathexis in the ego boundaries affected in various degress the feeling of awareness of parts of the somatic ego. The mental ego was similarly affected, rendering impossible various perceptive and executive functions serving reality adjustments. The volitional faculty, however, was less impaired as the ego boundaries under these circumstances contained the aggressive drives.

The following is a portion of a graphic description by this patient of one of her periodic crises.

> The frantic panic occurs when I feel I must continue, go on and on. I must feel that there is a definite termination of my working in view. There is a feeling of panic, palpitation, blinding. It actually blurs my vision and my head feels closed in and smaller when I am near a person for whom I feel aggression, and at the same time, a feeling of clinging . . . . She mustn't leave me—but I must have the power to leave her. This is true of men as well—anyone upon whom I depend for a feeling of belonging. I feel real only when I'm close to someone— actually kissing them or holding their eyes with mine. But at the same time I want to run away for fear they will leave me first and I'll be alone, proven worthless, unlovable . . . . I hate them for seeing me as I am and playing on it. It seems torturous to me. I fear working in the office and I fear not working; it all seems outside of myself. I'm all walled in within myself and I must fight my way out groping to belong to reality. When I feel panicky the only thing that stops it is a feeling that I can leave whenever I want to . . . . Working at the office is reality; I try to keep it in the foreground, but it constantly slips, and I feel it is something that must continue, the same thing every day, day in and day out, and I want to get away from it, to run to my own room, to

have the whole day to myself, to belong to someone who will take care of me. The end I seem to wait for is the being part of someone else to have strength to go on. Alone I need constant bolstering. As soon as I feel very much alone I have a feeling of something being torn out of me: an emptiness and a pulling, missing a heartbeat, a feeling in my diaphragm. It is a fear that now that I am alone I will lose control, things will happen to me, and I will be powerless to cry out.

This patient did not, unlike some others, accept the anhedonia. She resisted it, was aware only of tension and fear, and seemed to seek objects avidly. Each time, anxiety compelled her to retrace her steps. Analysis gradually made her aware of her lack of genuine interest in and feeling toward people. During crises she had to struggle to remain in contact with reality. The anhedonia was most clearly revealed in sexual intercourse. The nearest approximation to pleasure was the anticipation of closeness, reaching its peak in kissing; she remained completely frigid genitally. Her first genital orgasm was induced by a cannibalistic fantasy. When positive pleasure appeared, it revealed both the fixation and the defense against it which had resulted in anhedonia.

In her ambivalence and her cannibalistic fantasies accompanied by pain and tension about her mouth and teeth, this patient bears a striking resemblance to the cases of melancholia described by Abraham (1924) and Jacobson (1943). Abraham's patients had all suffered a double disappointment in their love for mother and father. The childhood history of his patients revealed a "primal depression" at the height of the oedipal struggle. This patient was not predominantly depressed. Her disappointment was chiefly in her mother, in the preoedipal period. Her childhood history revealed a primal detachment, or anhedonia.

Summary

Anhedonia, a lack of conscious pleasure, is presented as a clinical entity. This state is traced to its antecedents—a series of defensive reactions following very early and fairly specific traumata. The patients studied had schizoid characters. Attempts to establish object relationships result in a more or less stable state of anhedonia with periodic crises which threaten or terminate it. An economic and structural hypothesis, corresponding to the phenomenology, is presented. The genetic sequence is: pathogenic stimuli—oral-narcissistic fixation (first defense)—distance mechanism (secondary defense stabilizing the fixation)—anhedonia.

Additional Reading

M. Masud R. Khan. Clinical aspects of the schizoid personality; affects and technique. *International Journal of Psycho-Analysis*, 1960 41:430–437.

Chapter 9

A Deterrent in the Study and Practice of Medicine*

Clinical material and formulations are presented in this paper in an attempt to illuminate some difficulties inhibiting the study and practice of medicine. The difficulties are related to certain unconscious meanings of this discipline. These meanings stem from the normal modulations and pathological expressions of the broad instinctual roots of personality, as obviously they affect the choices of other vocations and professions as well. However, the difficulties which concern us here derive from specific instinctual drives and their modifiers only as they find expression in the studies and practices of medical discipline.

Which special instincts and instinctual derivatives may impel one to study and practice medicine? As a medical student, Freud wrote wittily to a school friend: "I have enrolled in another laboratory. Here I am preparing myself for my real profession to torture animals or to torment people. I come to favor more and more the first term of this alternative" (1897–1902, p. 16, n.2). Fifty years later he compressed some of the major determinants into a few sentences: "I became a doctor through being compelled to deviate from my original purpose. I have no knowledge of having had any craving in my childhood to succor suffering humanity. My innate sadistic disposition was not a very strong one, so that I had no need to develop this one of its derivatives. Nor did I ever play the 'doctor game'; my infantile curiosity evidently chose other paths" (1927, p. 253). Thus Freud stressed sadism and its transformation

*Originally published in the *Psychoanalytic Quarterly,* 1953, 22:381–412.

into compassion; and also infantile scoptophilia. And he cautioned: "It is not greatly to the advantage of patients if their physician's therapeutic interest has too marked an emotional emphasis. They are best helped if he carries out his task coolly and, so far as possible, with precision." Elsewhere he similarly advised analysts in training to observe their patients with the coolness of a sugeon (1912, p. 115).

Simmel (1926) followed up on Freud's observation. Analyzing the "doctor game," he found that it expressed the Oedipus complex and anxieties from primal scene fantasies, including the important scoptophilic component; also, that the acting out was propelled by the forces of the repetition compulsion. He equated the neurotic countertransference in the psychology of physicians with playing the "doctor game" and showed how it interfered with analytic practice.

Simmel's study did not include psychoanalytic physicians and students, though the basic principles of countertransference apply to all physicians. Simmel pointed out two related difficulties which apply to all neurotic physicians and students of medicine: (1) failing to develop a countertransference that permits a flexible distance from their patient, they tend to regress to one of excessive identification; (2) because of the taboo of the epistemophilic impulse, nurtured by the incest taboo, they cannot see. As a result of both difficulties, they cannot observe, but must act. Another dilemma concerns practitioners who in their professional attitude regress to viewing illness as the introjected parental substitute which is symbolized as excrement. To these the symbol is replaced by money, feces, upon which they displace the whole incestuous significance of their patients. This results in a taboo which prevents the physician from receiving money directly from the patients if he himself is to remain well or free from a sense of guilt. He avoids an inhibition in his work at the cost of an inhibition in being adequately paid for his services. Simmel drew a comparison between the "doctor game" of children and the transference of adults to the doctor during treatment and proved that the conclusion is justified that "the same instinctual impulse may make a given individual into a physician or a patient" (p. 476). This leads to the conclusion that the psychogenesis of the choice of the choice of the profession of medicine in an individual is a repetition of its phylogenesis, a fact made familiar through the researches of Róheim. Simmel quoted Róheim (1945) on the sublimation of sadistic instincts after the magician became the medicine man of primitive races. The magician's primal crime, incorporation of the parent substitute, was transformed into an excremental symbol or substance which caused disease and which must be ejected in order that the patient might recover.

Nunberg (1938b) stresses the possibility that a disturbance in professional efficiency may result from failure to relinquish the infantile fantasy of magical omnipotence, with a consequent temptation for the doctor to be pressed into the role allotted him by the patient. Nunberg relates excessive identification with patients to a feeling of guilt. He states that a healthy determinant for the practice of medicine is identification with the sick because every doctor has had the experience of having been a patient himself. He calls introjection of the parent substitute as the substance which caused disease demonic incorporation, and he speaks of healing as ejection or countermagic. Healing is also reincorporation, in sublimated form, on the level of genital libido. The patient, considering the physician a magician, unconsciously sees him in the role of a mother as well as of a father. The physician gladly accepts the role, unaware of his unconscious childhood wish to create new life and to bring children into the world. This wish is symbolized by the caduceus, the bisexual snake, connoting rebirth after death in sickness.

Lewin (1946a) shows the various ways in which medical education and the usual procedures in practice lend themselves to the normal transformations of such potentially disturbing phenomena as the patient's and the doctor's narcissism and primitive aggressive drives, and the doctor's craving for the ideal compliant patient, the cadaver. According to Lewin the cadaver represents the embodiment of all those preclinical basic sciences which deal with inanimate physical and chemical forces and substances, dead specimens and so forth. He does not discuss situations in which the countertransference becomes a neurosis, as exemplified in the failure to sublimate necrophilic fantasies. In the present study such situations and fantasies constitute the important starting points.

In his paper on necrophilia, Brill's (1941) clinical material deals primarily not with actual perverse behavior but with fantasies which he calls symbolic necrophilia, or sexual love for a dead body. From his review of the literature and the three cases he cites, two of which are his own, he describes the following basic phenomenology: a strong mother or grandmother fixation; fear of her death and the overcoming of that fear; aims of intercourse and mutilation of breast or body; vulturism; an inordinate craving for dermal contact; sadomasochism. The clarity of one of Brill's cases illustrates and corroborates my findings. It is the history of a man who became totally blind at four. He sought treatment because he had a strong craving to act out some of the aforementioned wishes with a cadaver. He had an especially strong craving to wallow in carrion. Taken with my findings, Brill's material contains illuminating suggestions for further understanding in terms of ego and superego defects. Brill mentions them, but his discussion is limited exclusively to the analysis of the id. He states that perversion is nothing but a magnified manifestation of infantile sexuality—a result of consti· tution and fate. The constitution of his patient is, of course, the sum of the erotogenic zones including the skin, and, in this instance, the fate is his blindness. However, Brill's discussion of the effects of that fate, though it is comprehensive, is limited to the patient's sexual development.

Besides these general observations and formulations which serve to orient us, the psychoanalytic literature contains only a few passing fragments of case reports referring to important difficulties in the study and practice of medicine. An exception is the literature on analytic countertransference, but here too the clinical excerpts are meager compared to the discussion of principles. A few brief remarks relate to our subject: Freud's (1927) reference to resistance toward sexuality among physicians; Glover's (1927) observation on the aversion of physicians to treating venereal diseases; an interesting bit of analysis by Jones (1911, p. 102) of a physician who placed a rigid stethoscope on his desk between himself and his patients; and Schmideberg's (1942) reference to a patient who wished to become a doctor in order to witness accidents, and another study (1930) in which she refers to the origin of surgery as possibly stemming from mutilation in connection with penitence. Henry H. Hart in a personal communication tells of a physician who, as a medical student, fainted in a urological clinic at the sight of penises exposed for treatment of a venereal disease, thus expressing passive homosexual and feminine wishes.

Kempner (1925) reported on a woman medical student whose oral-sadistic disposition led to her choice of profession. The orality and her identifications also produced an intestinal neurosis. The underlying psychopathology stressed was the orality and penis envy. The object of the paper was to demonstrate this orality; it is not clear, however, why the disturbance in identification and consequent neurosis affected her love relationships but not her professional activities.

Ernst Blum (1926) included in his data a medical student who equated intellectual attainment with potency and examination with birth and rebirth. There is a striking quotation from a woman medical student-patient who used the title of Rank's book, *The Trauma of Birth*—which she had not read—to describe her "finding a new self after graduation." Blum refers to pubertal initiation rites which symbolize the excision of organs and their replacement by new and maturer ones. He cites the interesting examples of a young man who had all his teeth extracted before an examination and a pre-examination epidemic of appendicitis in a school of fifty pupils. He equates the examination fear with castration fear and the appendectomies with symbolic fear of birth and ritualistic initiation of rebirth.

Deri (1942) described a male medical student whose wakefulness was part of a hostile identification with his physician-father. This identification interfered with his study of medicine to the point of his having to give it up. He then identified instead with his stepfather and followed the stepfather's profession.

I begin with a diagnostic interview which contains most of the significant phenomena in sharp outline:

Case A

A young physician just starting to practice was seen in connection with his application to work in a clinic. His record at college had been outstanding, but in medical school his marks fluctuated considerably. For two years he was in psychotherapy because of disturbing consequences of an attachment to a girl whom he labeled as a nymphomaniac and from whom he could not separate without the assistance of the therapist, who was a woman. When I saw him, he was in the process of separating from another girl, and felt it was now easier to do this as a result of the help he had received. Presumably, he had no difficulty with his duties as an intern, but he believed that the hospital authorities were exploiting the interns and were not interested in their education. When asked what branch of medicine particularly attracted or repelled him, he said he like medicine and pediatrics, but was especially repelled by gynecologists. They were hypocrites because, though they knew their patients only gynecologically, they often addressed them as "dear" or "dearie." None of his letters of reference came from faculty members of the medical school or executive officers of the hospital where he had been an intern, although this was suggested in the application and was the custom. He explained that the custom seemed to him meaningless, as no faculty member ever really knows a student. It was noted that both his letters of character reference were from women: his therapist, and a professional friend of his family.

To summarize, this physician encountered intellectual difficulties in medical school, though he had done exceptionally well in college. He was beginning to meet obstacles in his professional studies and contacts. Obviously related to these obstacles was another set of concurrent difficulties. He showed a compulsion to flee from women, who seemed to cling to him so overpoweringly that he needed the aid of another woman (the therapist) to free himself. It seemed to him that women could know him and could educate him better than men, who, moreover, tended to exploit him. But to know women was also to fear them because of their holding power, and, if one would avoid hypocrisy, to dislike them as well. In other words, he had an ambivalent attitude toward women, in which the hostile component was dominant, with an intimation of a feminine identification.

A conclusion suggested itself: perhaps there existed a connection between this patient's difficulties in intellectual mastery of the fundamentals of medicine and a possible coexistent feminine identification. For in both his professional and his heterosexual pursuits the obstacles that arose were similar in time of occurrence, in acuteness, in incongruity, and in irrationality. It is therefore not illogical to suspect a dynamic relationship between the two areas.

Case B

A first-year medical student came to analysis because he was unable to concentrate on or remember what he studied. He was depressed and despondent, and contemplated quitting medical school. These events were preceded by his decision to break with his girl. This he rationalized by supposing that she would not wait to marry him until he became economically self-sufficient, though she had never said so; and by saying that he was too proud to take any financial assistance from either family. His occasional evening snacks of milk and cake with the girl's brother and father were a more unmixed pleasure to him than was the girl herself. She was of a "good family," which meant that he might only "pet" with her, though after his depression and despondency lifted he could have fairly enjoyable sexual intercourse with girls of lower social and economic levels.

He despised his mother for her immaturity and frivolousness. His feeling for his father, a gentle but rather ineffectual man, was of friendliness and compassion, but not of intimacy. The one to whom he was closest and for whom he felt most respect was the maternal grandmother, the best-defined character and main financial support of the family, who had always lived closely with them. This matriarchal structure extended further to the great-grandmother, who had also lived with them until he was about ten.

He felt particularly hostile toward the great-grandmother who, according to the patient, dominated the family by her hypochondriasis. Memories from this early period disturbed him. They included the visits of doctors who took her pulse and, as he believed, appeased her, since he felt there was nothing the matter with her. He had decided he would not like to be that kind of doctor; he did not respect men who did that kind of work, as he did not respect such patients, who, however, stood for a larger group of women than he was aware. For such types as the wealthy matriarchal grandmother he had a measure of respect because of their power, though he had striven hard to become independent of her. He associated warmth and affection with lower-class women only;

these he could command but not marry. For the rest, such as his mother and "respectable" girls from his own social background, he felt hostility and a thinly disguised contempt. His idea of a real doctor was a surgeon who could do a major operation, such as a leg amputation.

With his classmates he was shy, as he had been in the army, where he kept to himself, was teased occasionally, and reacted aggressively, In the dissecting room he let the other members of the team take a more active role. He felt it was hard to adjust to the new subject matter. As an undergraduate he especially enjoyed the study of physical sciences because he could think out solutions to problems. In his medical studies this seemed less important. Anatomy, for example, was something he could not master intellectually, as he had the physical sciences in college. One somehow had to absorb it and be absorbed by it, he believed, merely by a feeling of closeness. Both processes seemed strange and frightening to him. At the same time he was becoming aware that his disturbed feelings about understanding medical subjects and about treating patients came from the fact that he would have to get into close contact with people. Once, discussing his work in the dissecting room, he made a slip, referring to the male cadaver they were dissecting as "she." He had several daydreams of working more actively in the anatomy laboratory. In all these the cadaver was a woman and the dissection involved the breast.

Following his second year, he volunteered to work in a hospital during the summer. His work included drawing samples of blood for chemical testing. He mastered his anticipatory anxiety and did his work satisfactorily. After his depression lifted he spoke hopefully of the possibility of mastering the clinical subjects as in college he enjoyed mastering the dead subjects of the physical sciences. He had less anxiety about working with female patients. During this phase it was possible to observe his predepressive personality. He was somewhat shy and reserved with classmates of his own sex. tended to address men in authoritative positions as "Sir," and found it easy to approach girls. Though very wary of meeting girls of his own class lest they get serious too quickly, he could easily approach girls at bars and wasted no time before having sexual relations with them. He had no potency difficulties, though occasionally he suffered from retarded ejaculation.

This patient's difficulty with the study of medicine appeared at the point of transition between the pleasurable mastery of the inanimate sciences and the fear of having to confront patients. The problem was to master the subject matter of his study which was undergoing a change; it seemed alive and dead at the same time. Such mastery could be attained only by closeness, incorporation, and assimilation. In the dissecting room this was felt as the incorporation of the cadaver as object. Anxiety and depression appeared with the growing awareness that this had already been experienced by him before: namely, that in some ways he was one with the "dead" mother—dead in the unconscious sense of being unresponsive, uninterested, withdrawn, and cold yet clinging. He conceived of his mother and his great-grandmother as being frivolous, controlling in an infantile way, essentially weak, and unable to give support. Though he dislike them, he had unconsciously identified with them or, more exactly, with a caricature of them. Though quite enterprising, painstaking, and capable of initiating activities and contacts, he appeared somewhat effeminate, was shy, felt inferior, disliked himself, and had a depressive tinge in his personality. At first, it seemed as if his moods of depression and anxiety followed the separation from his girl. Closer scrutiny, however, showed that the separation was deliberate, though rationalized, and was followed by relief. It was indeed a symbolic acting out of breaking union with the "dead" mother, an act of undoing. It was an attempt also to dispel a feeling of unreality. The attainment of a deeper sense of reality following the work of mourning was noted by Lewin (1950). This patient unconsciously devised a separation to cure a depression stemming from his medical studies. The depression was due to a new incorporation in line with his character, which, though fairly stable, was chronically depressive. Ablation of the breast symbolized his birth into freedom; for thus he himself was, by part-object identification with the breast, freed from his mother.

Case C

A general practitioner in his early thirties was not aware that he was too distant with most of his patients and too intimate with a few. The distance was part of a chronic dream state in which he lived. Everything he knew and did seemed to him vague and hazy. He could not retain details, theoretical or practical. Such matters as hospital arrangements and applications, as well as some rather customary procedures, he was content to know about in a general way. His work was routine, sketchy, and mediocre; not deliberate, thoughtful, or distinguished by any feelings of pleasure or of competency.

In medical school, his studies also had seemed to him unreal and hazy, and his effort inadequate. He did not have the strength to penetrate as deeply as he should because he had images of phallic inadequacy and because his incestuously tinged epistemophilic urge was inhibited. A further cause was a pathological type of optimism, derived from identification and expressed as, "I don't have to know, mother knows, and will take care that I pass the examination." At one point he recognized that the analysis was helping him give up his identification with his mother. He could see some aspects of his behavior clearly and sharply. At about the same time he reported that he watched a hemorrhoidectomy at the hospital. He said, "It seemed very simple. I saw no need for all the fuss. You just expose, clamp, tie, and cut off. Analysis is not so complicated either. Saying this gives me a pleasant taste in my mouth." Elaborating, he said that it seemed to him that the operation removed a slice of the buttock. This was a condensation of two images: detachment from the breast and severing the vascular connection, the umbilical cord, which was for him, at least in part, accomplished by using the mouth to bite one's way out, so to speak.

He felt close to his mother, sister, and wife, in a strange way. He felt as one of them, moved more among them than among men in the family, but he took them for granted and ordered them about. His comments about his father and brother were more sharply etched, but he was more removed from them. He felt superior to them, yet envied them their matter-of-factness in contrast to his dreamy, hazy images of himself and his life. His attachment to the women in the family had a mixture of libidinal and aggressive elements, paralleling his sexual play with girls, with whom possessiveness, oral satisfaction, the breast, and dermal contacts in particular were the all-important elements. While a medical student he demonstrated to his sister the method of breast palpation for the diagnosis of cancer. Later, when his sister was about to give birth, he thought his mother wanted him to know about every contraction and be present at the delivery. He desisted, however, because his sister "had a competent obstetrician." It did not occur to him that there are certain things brothers do not do, even though they are doctors. He was puzzled as he felt he understood what the women in the family were thinking or wished him to do, but, on the other hand, his mother usually spoke to his wife first and the messages were relayed to him. It was as if he were being protected, as if he could not be let in on the secrets of the adults. He was either one of the women or a child. In his unconscious he was both, with the child symbolized by the breast or phallus.

As an expression of his anger because they were moving from the house where he was born, he played a joke on his mother. While she was busying herself arranging various jars of preserves and homemade wines, he urinated into one of them and, making his father an accomplice, asked her to sample it. This joke, like a dream, represented a condensation of several important elements: his phallic identification with the children in the hospital, who impressed him chiefly as "urinators"; punishment for an oral frustration by oral and urinary aggression; and identification with his father, a dependent, depressive character given to suicidal threats. The mother appeared as the stronger person. The patient often told about her forcing food on everyone and her habit of stuffing the icebox to capacity. He liked to use the double entendre for breast feeding as "a bust in the mouth." Because we know the mechanism of identification, so important for ego maturation, is the result of an incorporative act, we recognize that for one to regard being fed as an aggressive act perpetrated upon him is to be fixated very early in an ambivalence with a resulting serious incapacity for adequate identification. One of the best examples is the incapacity to resolve the Oedipus complex.

In working through his problems of vagueness he remarked: "At school, I felt it was enough to be just vaguely aware so as to be able to write 400 words about it." His associations were: "The 400 living on Park Avenue," and of envying a boy who entered the elevator with him just before the analytic hour. In questioning the elevator man, the boy seemed to be definite and poised. Obviously the patient wished to be that boy, the analyst's boy. This reminded him of a dream he had had the night before: "A large house burned down; it was my folks' home. My mother was in the house. I'm looking through heaps of ashes." His associations led to feelings of guilt about his curiosity and about a compulsion to see the analyst's home in the country; he had fleeting thoughts about his wife's dying in an automobile accident and her resemblance to his mother. He now recalled another detail of the dream: he was using a stick to poke around in the ashes. He recalled scenes of ruins and his inability to make distinctions, for example, between the Rhone and the Seine rivers, or the relationship between France and Spain. After mentioning many areas—politics, art, and so forth—he said, "I am chagrined, I have no clearly defined facts at my fingertips. It is not good for a physician not to know the facts"—obviously the facts of life. Associations to "large house" were: big penis, envy of his father's penis, concern about his own small penis, and of losing his penis; identification with and aggression toward little girls. There were also primal-scene images confused with death scenes; for example, he showed confusion between "lay" and "lied" in a casket, and expressed both a wish to die in a big house and a fear lest he die before he was mature. Besides the castration anxiety in these primal scene fantasies we note confusion between male and femal, between sexual acts or birth and death, and wishes for and fears of rebirth, the last representing the struggle over breaking with his feminine identification.

The pleasure of loitering amidst ruins, we have learned to recognize from this patient and from other patients, is a disguise for the mixed pleasure of being close to the "dead" mother and at the same time feeling free from her. It is noteworthy that the symbols for the clutching and cold mother are liquids or semisolids, like water, weeds, clay, quicksand, or ashes. The symbols for the dead mother who gave up or gave birth to her child are solid, like stone walls, rocks, mountains. These give footing and support as well as freedom of motion. Both sets of symbols are disguises for necrophilic fantasies, which basically represent wishes for separation as well as for union.

We can now connect the patient's professional inhibitions with the vagueness that resulted from primal-scene anxieties, including epistemophilic anxiety. We find that his self-image is confused with his image of his mother. He also visualizes himself as breast and phallus, and he has a wish to be reborn in the masculine image.

Case D

A first-year medical student was afraid of competing with the other members of his class whom he considered older and better qualified than he. He was correct only in the sense that he was aware of his own emotional immaturity. Although he had been a good student at college, he failed several of the monthly tests in anatomy. His fear mounted as he faced the final examinations, which he passed with one exception. He failed but finally passed in chemistry under the following circumstances. He came late the morning of the final examination. He was so upset when he faced the chemistry instuctor, who was generally regarded as a bully and whom he especially feared, that he could not follow the instructions for the test, and failed. In the fall he was adequately prepared for re-examination. The apparatus was set up by another instructor. While working on a urine analysis, the patient sniffed a bit of the vapor from a reagent bottle he was using. It was a solution of cyanide salt. He became panicky, feared for his life, wondered about seeing a doctor, and had visions of himself dead on the autopsy table of the hospital. He recalled a lecture in toxicology in which the fearsome instructor told about the death of a man in a hotel room from odors remaining after fumigation. As a result he was unable to finish his work and failed his re-examination. The dean of the school, whom he regarded as kind and fatherly, gave him another chance without even listening to his explanation. He finally passed a second re-examination which was given by a very friendly old professor.

The following year he came into analysis because of a speech phobia which produced, when he spoke, a peculiar, affectless tachylalia. After a time he made a transference improvement in his speech. When he was asked to describe his improvement, he said, "Somehow I have no fears talking to you. Then I talk slowly and with life in my voice. Now, when I'm outside of here and have to speak, I put myself in my mind under a kind of bell jar, like the one you put a microscope under, and imagine myself in your consultation room. In that atmosphere, I can talk without fear." If we now add that in his fantasies he loved to talk and impress audiences, and that a frequent synonym of his for speech was a "lethal spray," we can see a link between the lethal gas-filled hotel room of his examination panic and the benign enclosure of his counterphobic fantasy, the bell jar. In the first instance he was in a panic about getting deeper into his medical studies, at the peril of his life, because of his guilt about looking at and knowing the human body. The exaggerated fear of the rough instructor completes the acting out of primal-scene anxiety with particular reference to punishment for infantile scoptophilia at the hands of a severe father image. But the punishment by death for oedipal guilt is merged with the idea of protection or sleep in a havenlike enclosure, symbolic of the mother.

We note the equation of being inside a gas-filled room with being a cadaver on the dissecting table. The image of oedipal phallic castration becomes confluent with that of maternal separation. The body as phallus merges and interchanges with the body as embryo-breast. Lethal gas represents the primal-scene fantasy of phallic functioning as well as the image of an orally aggressive function of the breast.

The patient was the second sibling. The first died in infancy from an infectious diarrhea. As a result of this our patient was anxiously nursed for eighteen months. Weaning from his mother was very difficult, evidenced by attacks of anorexia and diarrhea at the outset of his schooling.

The breast as an orally aggressive organ, with a powerful mouth threatening to incorporate, was visualized by him as having a concave surface (a variation of the dream screen [Lewin, 1946b]), looking like the shell of an acorn and exerting strong suction. Accordingly, he fancied that strong oral and muscular activity was required on the part of the infant to counteract this pull. The bell jar was thus the transformation of the setting of the primal scene, the womb, the abdomen, and the breast, in the shape of an acorn shell. Ultimately it represented the image of the good breast and the image of phallic identification with the protecting father. His first interests in medical specialization were pediatrics and gastroenterology.

This patient's epistemophilic inhibition was compensated for by a wish to exihibit what he did know. The inhibition of intellectual curiosity or potency was compensated for by a strong exhibitionistic desire expressed through speech, which was also felt to be lethally aggressive. The speech phobia aimed at warding off the consequences of such aggression.

In the transference he made from the counterphobic fantasy the step which Simmel's (1926) female patient made in playing the doctor game: the step from feminine sadomasochism to childlike dependence upon a good father. This marks an advance in the following ways. His scoptophilic guilt is removed; he can see all minutiae as through a microscope. Not fearing castration, he has less need for compensatory exhibitionism and aggression. His words are therefore not lethal and he need not fear them, as he did not fear identification with the doctor's instrument (microscope-phallus). Another advance is that looking is now also an ego and superego function, integrated with guiding motility, in contrast to the phobic fantasy in which it is entirely a forbidden id manifestation, punishable by immobilization, felt as death or sleep.

This patient has, in common with almost all the others, fantasies or dreams about death. They represent, as in Simmel's patient, what he calls "coming to grief in the Oedipus conflict over the synthesis (confluence) of her pregenital and genital libidinal tendencies" (p. 477). We may add that libido may become reattached in a narcissistic way to the id or to the mother (the primary source of libido). Either cathexis is regressive and to the ego spells death. Similarly, as the ego emerges by "finding" itself as an object and separating from the mother, the evolution is feared as the death of both mother and self. Through analysis the patient was able to overcome this confluence of libidinal tendencies. In becoming a successful pediatrician, he was able to sublimate his primary identification and to identify with the analyst as the good father.

Case E

A surgeon of 38, young-looking and effeminate, was troubled by depressive moods, disturbances of potency, and difficulties in his work. His hands trembled while he operated, he was overly anxious about inhalation anesthesia, too often he thought of the emergency procedure of tracheotomy, and he tended to substitute medical procedures for surgical ones. Usually he failed to charge adequate fees, but occasionally overcharged. In accepting patients referred to him by two older colleagues, he felt unduly bound and constrained by their directives, and complained that he had "no personal practice."

His father, who had died fifteen years before, had been a successful surgeon, harsh and punitive toward all members of the family and often ruthless in his dealings with people. His mother was long-suffering and submissive, anxious, ineffectual, and subject to periods of depression. An early memory was of falling out of his crib and down an embankment; his mother was away, and a man nearby had his back turned and offered no help. A later memory was of his father snapping a picture of him in the woods defecating. Another was of a struggle with the anesthetist before his tonsillectomy at age seven or eight. His father had brought him to the hospital by a ruse. Somewhat later, memories related to his mother and blood-soaked underclothes, suggesting menstruation or abortion. Pleasant memories were about his mother cooking, his grandmother's quaint old world-dishes, and his mother's fondness for a bobtailed female cat. As a boy he was not allowed to use roller skates and first learned to ride a bicycle at age 21. In college he felt lost, was self-conscious about his poor skin, and thought he had a small penis. He blamed his parents for depriving him of stamina.

He practiced masturbation in late adolescence. He had no sexual relations before marriage at age 25. His wife appealed to him in an unusual way; she was shy, unaggressive, and looked more boyish than feminine. By courting her he could prove to her more feminine and successful sister and to the girl herself that her type need not be considered a failure, destined to spinsterhood. Another attraction was that her parents were warmer people than his. His narcissistic identification with his wife was motivated among other factors by the urge to rivalry with his own sister, older by four years and more aggressive. He enjoyed shopping for food and waiting on his wife. She had a depressive character and was subject to frequent respiratory infections. She worked as a secretary, first from necessity and later by choice. Their sexual life was first plagued by his occasional premature ejaculations, and gradually grew worse. Soon after the birth of their child there was very little sexual activity. He withdrew emotionally from his wife, but had no sexual interest in other women. With the aid of a maid, the care of his 7-year-old daughter was mainly his responsibility and consisted mostly of nurturing or mothering. With the women in his family he was very distant and cold. He never spoke of them except when they intruded themselves upon his attention, and then he would try to avoid them. His general manner, his passive masochistic attitudes, indicated that these women were part of him, but it was as if this part of him were cold and dead and threatened to invade the rest of him. He acted this out in life but could not tolerate being conscious of it.

During phases of positive transference his potency would improve. One occasion, however, was different. The surface reason he gave seemed curious, but its meaning soon became evident. His wife decided to undergo an operation for a painful foot condition rather than accept longer, conservative nonoperative treatment. It seemed to him that through this courageous decision she came to life. She was going to submit to an operation by a surgeon who was gentle and conservative, and not be like his mother who submitted to his brutal father, the surgeon, who must have hurt her sexually as he did in other ways. By this one important decision, his wife stepped out of the role of substitute for his incestuous love object. In addition, her decision meant to him that she had determined to eliminate, like the medieval exorcising of the devil, the illness they had in common, an illness compounded of depression and lethargy suggestive of lifelessness, which acted as an additional barrier to closeness. The effect of her decision, however, was not long-lasting.

This experience also served to express his dependence upon the analyst's activity. When he was active outside the analytic hours, he was doing his "homework" for the analyst-father. For a period he busied himself with thoughts of being a psychiatrist. This identification did not last. It could not master his fear of the analyst because of his deep hostility and envy, expressed in various jokes and sarcasm about analysts; nor could he identify with the analyst when he visualized him as a maternal figure who worked at home and was spared the battles among men in the external world, such as those of surgeons for hospital privileges and status. Identification failed because of the combination of deep hostile wishes and because the approach was passive and therefore dangerous. This same approach determined one of his forms of resistance. He attempted to entertain the analyst and seduce him into giving direct advice about various problems in his daily practice. He wanted to live out the experience of being indulged by a good father, rather than express in transference his feelings about a rejecting father. At the same time, he knew that he would be frustrated by not being given direct answers. Thus he would live out the rejection in a milder form, a rejection partly libidinized, rather than encounter the full wrath of his father.

The wish to be fed with the possibilities of satisfaction and disappointment, which in effect he expressed in transference, was a repetition of a wish to be adequately cared for. This wish, in its full sense, was originally denied at the maternal source. In his formative years, his father was too completely absorbed in his work and was not close enough to his son to contribute positively or to neutralize the effects of his mother's influence. From the mother's closeness he retained, as we saw, the unusual interest in food, to the extent of liking to market for his own family. This close tie offered him anxious overprotection and produced in part what he called the deprivation of his stamina. We may recall his earliest memory of falling out of his crib and down an embankment. His mother was absent and the man standing by turned his back on him. The combination of the effects of aggressive feeling, anxious overprotection, and inadequate real protection, seems to have been a major cause of his disturbed capacity for identification.

Both parents were part of him in a strange way, like an encapsulated disease, at times pleasurably affecting all of him in a benign way, and at other times threatening to envelop him completely and dangerously. This conclusion was derived from the following striking reaction in the transference. At certain times, after some words were spoken by the analyst, he would assume a distant and drowsy appearance. On occasion he would resist this state by propping himself up higher on the couch, or by sitting up, or by suggesting that the analyst speak to him or engage in conversation. It seemed that speaking to him promoted and at the same time combated the drowsy state. This state denoted the feeling of encapsulation as pleasurable or dangerous. In the same mood he would enter into ruminations such as these: "How does it feel to be dead? . . . How many years more have I got to live? . . . In so many years more I should be the age of my father when he died. . . . How awful and undignified the body appears at autopsy, the nostrils stuffed with cotton and the penis tied off with a piece of gauze . . . ."

The themes of the blocked nostrils, suggesting dyspnea and death, and of the dead or castrated penis appeared in other forms. Subject to frequent colds, and once having had a nasal polyp removed, he had an acute exacerbation of nasal congestion when the analyst was absent for a few days. He was certain that he had a new polyp, visualized it as a round, cystlike mass which acted as a valve shutting off his expiration. He wished to have it removed surgically, or at least to have his antrum irrigated. The laryngologist he consulted saw no indication for either procedure. To prove that he had what he called a real congestion, he brought with him to the analyst's office a little bottle containing an astringent for the nasal mucosa, but forgot to bring the medicine dropper. He wondered whether the analyst might have one among his drug samples. He was surprised to find an appreciable clearing of his nasal congestion by the end of the analytic session.

The patient's identification with his dead father in these fantasies is evident. The analyst's absence was a similar death. But, in addition, he had fearful thoughts about the possibility of someone's being buried while deeply asleep and then dying from suffocation. Similarly, he had inordinate fears of inhalation anesthesia, frequently checking the anesthesia unit and the emergency tracheotomy instruments. Thus, he feared his own death would result from the death of his father and father substitute. His pent-up rage and hostility against his father was most difficult for him to express. One recognized it only from glimpses of his angry facial expression when he spoke of his father's taking a humiliating picture of him, deceiving him about his own tonsillectomy, and mistreating his mother.

But the identification with the parent who leaves or dies was determined by more than the guilty fear of retaliation from the father. The analyst also represented the mother, as shown above. This relationship contained a paradoxical double fear of death: the

one, from abandonment; the other, from great closeness or anticipation of great closeness. It was felt as olfactory or respiratory
incorporation, choking, and an inability to give up or exhale. The
organs which he feared would choke the breath and life out of him
were the breast and penis. It was obviously not solely the factor of
mechanical obstruction to respiration that was feared. In any event,
death in realistic terms was not feared as it was not envisaged. What
was feared was a form of regressive, attenuated life. One's breath
was not one's own, and one could not get rid of that breath by
exhalation and inhale again for oneself. We might say that this
image represents the loss of self, expressed in respiratory language.
The fear of dying from being buried meant a fear of being
immobilized like an organ.

To recapitulate, we have shown some phenomenological and
affective expressions of part-object identification and some evidence
of the patient's identification with castrating and castrated individuals in his life. What follows will indicate some of the manifestations resulting from the confluence of pregenital and genital self-
images and identifications. It also shows the effects of this confluence
and the struggle to interpret it in his professional activities.

He had been at a loss regarding the type of practice to choose
after his internship. What forced him to decide quickly was his fear
of being drafted and killed: "It so happened that a residency
presented itself and it turned out to be the same as my father's,
surgery." It was really a deliberate unconscious choice to save his
life; in self-defense he turned to his father identification. With the
subsidence of his fear, he found it hard to follow his father's
specialty. He occasionally noticed a fine tremor of his hands during
an operation and felt embarrassed lest this be noticed. Some types
of surgery he would not attempt at all. Operations about the head
were too dangerous. The mind and the intellect were two expressions of potency by which he could identify with his father, whom
he resembled in being quite bright. But in the professional and
sexual sense he regarded his father as a killer and a castrator. He
could not do the same work; when he did, he identified instead with
the patients he operated upon. He indulged them and nursed them
as he wished he might be in the analysis. He feared for their death
by suffocation, as he feared any slight impairment in his own

breathing. Hence he could not operate on the thorax. When he thought he might be exposed by some of the results because he "could not reach far," his alternative was to turn to his father identification, to kill by wishes and thoughts. In his unconscious a surgeon was someone with a big phallus. Referring to himself as a surgeon, he called himself a piddler, adding that he "could not reach the end point," and that he had wet the bed till the age of 13. In other words, he had a small penis, like the patient attacked and castrated by the father-surgeon. In a similar fashion, his passive, masochistic dependence upon his father made it hard for him to be comfortable with patients referred to him by older surgeons. Because of such referrals, he complained he did not have a "personal practice." As he was chiefly identified with his patients, he could not carry out some of the procedures recommended because he had some question about their usefulness. For one thing, all the patients seemed to belong to the older surgeons, the father surrogates, as if they were the women in the family who all belonged to the father. He sometimes unwittingly referred to all patients, irrespective of their sex, as "she" or "it."

In characterizing himself as an inadequate surgeon or a piddler, he wanted to add, "I am not a real surgeon," instead of which he said, "I am not a breast surgeon." Unconsciously then, for him a real surgeon was a breast surgeon. They made more money than he did, that is, they had no inhibition about charging. There was one form of operation he liked to perform: draining and squeezing pus pockets and removing cysts. To an irrational degree he sought to have this type of operation performed on himself for the removal of a round cystic mass which he believed caused a "ball-valve" obstruction to his breathing. The allusions to the breast are clear enough, although the male genitalia are also suggested.

Let us turn to the episode of the analyst's absence, the patient's nasal congestion in anticipation of his return, and his wish for a medicine dropper. Such mucosal congestion in a passive receptive state is well known. But other events and facts from this context must be mentioned. The condition began just as or a little before the analyst left; it was exacerbated by his return. Furthermore, he wished the analyst to remove his congestion after the fashion of a laryngologist removing a polyp or a cyst. What caused his congestion in the first place? We learned that during the analyst's absence he met a woman, whom he described as the very active type, who hinted about her sexual frustration. In an objective manner he advised sexual gratification, but did not offer himself, the obvious object in her mind. In this connection he began to ruminate about death, about the possibility that people who apparently have ceased to breathe, but are not dead, might be buried. His associations turned to his wife. She was more attractive to him at the moment because she was more active in general and more giving to him. Yet he was fearful and did not let her go on this way. At this point, he added, "I have nothing to say, I want you to speak." What he meant was that he feared the oral incorporative aims of such women. They might devour him as actively as they fed him. The breast being a feeding and devouring organ for him, he regressed to the image and status of an attached organ, the breast. The analyst, through his benevolent talking or using of the medicine dropper, could then be in turn the liberator and remove him or help him bite his way out of the status of an organ, the breast, and thus help him to emerge as an organism. The acquired phallus would also function as a liberating scalpel.

He had a dream at this time: "A cat had a litter of kittens. I saw a cord hanging down, and it seemed as if she had eaten a part of it." He was reminded that when he was a small boy the family had a bobtailed cat; also of a maiden aunt with the same name. His mother was fond of the cat and was very much attached to Aunt Jackie. He thought the cord hung from the "bottom" or rectum and that it was eaten after birth. Vague memories of bloodstained clothes made him think of his mother's several abortions. When irrigating and draining pockets of infection in various parts of the body of a patient, he felt like an abortionist and the operation as an incestuous act. He felt he "killed the kid." Currently, he was puzzled by the fact that though he was generally timid and aloof, he felt pleased and elated "like a kid" when someone was sweet to him, said "please," or called him by his first name. He was then "pulled in." From this dream we learn that he sees himself as the aggressive father-surgeon who killed the child, and that he is also identified with the child. As the child, he is dead or asleep when separated from his mother, but is alive, elated, when pulled in and thus rein-corporated by the mother. In turn that state of closeness is feared, as is expressed by his general aloofness. Occasionally he has a critical need for more sudden separation. When it was suggested that the dream pointed to a shift toward seeing himself in the role of his father, albeit with feelings of guilt, he replied, "You want to push me out. I think I'm getting a hernia. This may require surgery. A delay may disclose that perhaps it is cancer." He had corrected me by pointing out that I failed to recognize that he was open below and might have something growing in his abdomen, like a pregnancy. In other words, he was still part of the mother-child unity, he was mother and child, and the problem of separation was still unsolved. In effect he was asking the analyst to put first things first. The father identification frightened him, and he therefore avoided doing major or difficult surgery. Realistically this was a serious matter, but psychologically the fear could be checked by the inhibition. On the other hand, the conflicts arising from the mother identification were more disturbing. This identification he attempted to resolve through acting out being a breast surgeon. Separation of the breast from the body would symbolize liberation of the child from oneness with the anxious, depressed, "dead" mother.

Describing his residency in surgery, he said that he had not known what it would be like before he entered into it. Referring to his inhibitions about operating, it did not seem real to him that he should be doing what his father had done. He was dreamy and tended to be resigned rather than aggressive.

That night he dreamed: "My child B died, and her brother; later I died. It took place in an operating room. Something that had to be fed to the patient from what looked like a soap dispenser, the kind I use in my office, ceased to work, and the patient died on the operating table."

Background for the dream included an impending visit from his mother, who had for some months been confined to her home because she was depressed. He did not want to be involved with her. He was annoyed and wished she were dead. Actually he had only one child, a girl. In his attitude toward her, he both identified her with himself and treated her as a sibling. Though he had realized it was a dream, he had walked into his child's room and looked at her. The soap dispenser in the dream, he said, was different from his. His contained white soap; in the dream it was yellowish, like urine. In association to his child's dying, he spoke about his anger at a woman patient upon whom he operated. The sinus which he had established for draining a bone abscess closed. He did not remove the infection, and she got no help. He wished she would die to cover up his mistake.

In this dream the patient is in the role of the father-surgeon-killer. We also see his inferiority and guilt in that impersonation. If the victim died both f elings would be abated. But the victim and the death are overdetermined. First it is the mother, the victim of the father's sexual operation, in accordance with the child's conception of the primal scene. Then it is the child as a boy, emasculated and killed in retribution for his oedipal wishes. The repetition of the "doctor game" in the dream, in accordance with his acting it out in his practice, is, as Simmel (1926) said, indicative of the failure or absence of an adequate identification with the father. That indicates that our subject's choice of profession was based on preoedipal fixations in which the repressed object, the mother, returns in the form of his patient. But the death of the mother has still another meaning. We learned from the dream background his wish to be separated from her; furthermore, the woman he operated upon was an asthmatic, and one of the aims of the operation was to relieve her of the asthma by creating a channel for draining the encapsulated infection. We find here all the elements for the operation of the *accoucheur*. Furthermore, the embryo also stands for the internal breast. Thus, the breast surgeon is the disguised obstetrician. Our patient plays the role, in doctor-game fashion, in turn, of the father, mother, and child-breast-phallus. Incidentally, in his fear lest his breathing be choked off, he resembles dynamically the asthmatic and the claustrophobic. In a case of claustrophobia, Lewin (1935) found that the patient was identified with the embryo on a basis of sibling hostility. These facts support an additional motivation, namely, identification with the hostile, sexually aggressive father or phallus.

Interesting corroboration is to be found in the patient's projections on the report of the Rorschach, Thematic Apperception, and Drawing tests:

> A recurrent theme is that of the two women "back-to-back" or "who have been torn apart." There is a good deal of variation in sexual

fantasy, with moments in which he conceives of his sexual equipment as exceedingly vulnerable and helpless, and other times when it seems like an instrument of aggressive prowess. Very often he projects a sense of "pained resignation," a feeling that the drives and tensions may be too overwhelming and "now it is a matter of giving up." This attitude of "resignation" [his own terms] is also used to describe the mother and may represent some kind of identification with her. And the sense of "depletion" extends to heterosexual relations where he negates the sexualized content and makes the lover a physician who has been unable to save his patient. In his response to card B.M.F., which symbolizes heterosexual relations, he states, "The guy is either tired or in despair. She's dead or drunk or dead-drunk. I have the feeling maybe it's a physician who tried very hard to save this woman. It's all over and he put so much in it, he feels depleted. Yet it looks like a young man and a young woman. There are books there and not the setting of acute illness that would end that way. It almost looks like a husband and wife."

His drawing of his Most Unpleasant Concept is an operating room and figures in surgical garb around a child whose mouth is wide open. He said, "It's myself and assistants. The child is bleeding on the table; it looks like Ku Klux Klan figures." Associating to these figures he related an experience when he was seven or eight. While traveling with his mother in the country during the Prohibition era, he spied a policeman on a motorcycle, whereupon his mother threw a bottle of whisky out of the car. The symbolic act indicates castration and weaning; the symbolic figures again point to father, mother, child-breast-phallus. His Most Pleasant Concept is a patient and an attending doctor with a big sun shining in the sky and labeled "Miracle Doctor." He said, "This is my patient, Sally Sunshine. She represents success."

This patient converted the aggression of his "primary identification" mostly into symptoms, and that of his secondary identification mostly into inhibitions, both of which affected his surgical work.

Discussion

In approaching their patients, the medical students and practitioners of our series had inhibitions, symptoms, and symptomatic acts directly related to their choice of profession. In general they were not able to maintain an optimal, flexible distance from their patients, being too close to some, too distant from others, and fluctuating from one extreme to the other with the same patient.

At closer range, the causal factor of the deterrent noted in all was that their typical patient was the projected mother, and the typical therapy was the ablation of the breast with which they were identified. The underlying aim was an attempt to complete the cathexis of their own ego, amounting to a cure of their ego defect, to "find" and "choose," as Tausk (1934) put it, or "bind," as Simmel (1926) expressed it, their narcissistic object and masculine ideal.* More precisely, the involvement of these patients with this task contained the raw material for the deterrent. It is possible, of course, for the healthy male, as was the case in certain of our patients after treatment, to resolve the fixation upon the "primary identification" by sublimation. Indeed, this accomplishment is a major prerequisite for mental health. When the sublimation is a stable one it becomes possible for it to mix in varying proportions with elements of the oedipal identification in determining voca- tional choice. In our patients the principal determinant in the choice of profession was the oedipal ideal. The secondary deter- minant, which became the deterrent, was the "primary identifica- tion." However, the oedipal expressions were relatively muted because they took the form of inhibitions and because the solution of the regressive conflict became prerequisite.

In the formative stages of the ego, the doctor served as the ego ideal, as well as being a means of satisfying id strivings. Doctors were actually though not always conscious ego ideals in the families of these patients, and were a determinant in the choice of medicine as a profession. But identification with them was impossible because of unsolved difficulties in the tie with an earlier ego ideal, the mother. The compulsion to solve them reactivated this regressive "primary identification" on the basis of part-object identification.

Neither of these identifications, which in our opinion approx- imate each other, is a true identification; rather, they are symbiotic fusions. Identification as a fundamental mechanism for psychosexu-

---

*This process of severing the highly cathected feminine self, symbolized by the breast, from the masculine with which it is confluent, and toward which it offers an incorporative threat, is comparable to one conception of circumcision, as described by Nunberg (1947), wherein the removal of the feminine component, the prepuce, serves the same purpose.

al, affective, and intellectual development, is an important function of the ego after it has evolved from the status of part-object and has "found" itself as total object. The ego has then a capacity for active incorporation and passive receiving of the role of another person, the essence of identification. Either capacity is aborted when the narcissistic object-finding experience is marked by traumata. We may say that there remains a fixation on the traumatic events of the time when the ego was being "born." Under these circumstances identification is rendered impossible. The necessary activity is not inherent in an ego that has not yet "found" itself; such activity is then felt to belong outside. The necessary passivity is then feared as a regression into the id, as a disappearance or a death.

We were impressed to find that most of these patients felt feeding simultaneously as a libidinal gratification and as an aggression—an attempt at reincorporation. It was a mixed traumatic experience. One consequence of this was the mobilization of aggression in the form of increased oral activity, general motility, and scoptophilia to master the danger of reincorporation. Insofar as identification presupposes relinquishment or transformation of aggressive energy, it was further rendered impossible, or could act only partially.

An interesting feature was the importance of scoptophilia, serving first as a partial sexual drive and then undergoing transformation as an ego component integrated into the service of motility. Motility was felt to be synonymous with birth or emergence of the differentiated self.

The conflict between ego regression and progression was reflected in necrophilic ruminations. Accordingly, the clinging mother promoted the one side of the conflict, and the birth-giving, or "dead" mother the other side. Both images were projected onto mother nature in the inanimate, in the forms of liquids and semisolids, on the one hand, and solids, on the other. An example of the latter was the enjoyment of scenes of ruins, accompanied by a state of elation and a feeling of being the lone master of the earth. These projections may affect the attitudes of the medical student toward the dead preclinical subjects and the cadaver, and ultimately determine whether his attitude toward his patients will be sublimated or neurotic.

Chapter 10

The Rebirth Motif in Homosexuality and Its Teleological Significance*

This paper reports on an additional syndrome (see Ch. 9 and Ch. 11) that derives from the incomplete dissolution of, or fixation upon, the primary identification (see Ch. 9) of the mother-child symbiosis. These syndromes may coexist in the same patient, as might be expected in view of their common roots. Several factors are common to all of them. There are distortions in ego functioning, especially in identification. Prominent are multiple part-object identifications with breast and phallus of the phallic mother and with her castrated body image. These part-self-images are cathected predominantly with destructive aggression and have passive incorporative aims in relation to the narcissistic ideal image of a total-self—the phallic mother. Noteworthy is failure in accomplishing the final phase of identification—assimilation. Attempted transitions from the self-image of an organ to that of a total organism are not felt as a gradual maturational process in terms of accretion and differentiation, but rather are felt (and feared) as sudden, cataclysmic emergence into a new and definitive state, strongly suggestive of the process of birth, in effect—rebirth.

Keeping these common factors in mind, I deem it useful to include here a very brief recapitulation of the theme of rebirth as it appears in the previous studies, in each of which it has a different form and significance. Incidentally, the term motif in the title was chosen because it is more generic than fantasy, inasmuch as the

---

*Originally published in the *International Journal of Psycho-Analysis*, 1956, 37:416–421.

latter, though clear in some cases, is in other cases more obscure and less recognizable by the patient as such.

In working through aspects of passivity, several patients who stuttered dwelt on the difficulties and futility of changing to a more active role. They indulged in wishful thinking akin to the proverbial jumping out of one's skin and becoming someone completely different. Their attitude called to mind a remark made to me by Dr. Martin Bergmann[1] about "patients who wish for a trade-in operation instead of a repair job." Inevitably there was much concern about the fate of the discarded self. One patient acted this out by recording his stuttering speech on a tape recorder. While listening to the tape he was able to speak quite fluently, "correcting" the stutterer's speech. Thus, externalization of his old self while yet keeping it within earshot was essential before he could be "reborn" in identification with his therapist. The same patient, in a similar context, stated that what he really needed was an earthquake, implying a rebirth wish as well as a wish for an induction with a higher degree of active energy.

The second syndrome (see Ch. 9) dealt with a special type of inhibition in the study and practice of medicine. The inhibition was traced to a need to break with important remnants of the primary identification. The medical analysand regarded his typical patient as the mother and the typical therapeutic procedure as an ablation of the breast, with which organ he was identified. This break, often accompanied by separation anxieties and agoraphobic reactions, was also experienced as a kind of birth, or rebirth.

The third syndrome (see Ch. 11) dealt with what was termed "agoraphilia"—that may be defined by its chief characteristics—a special fascination for the out-of-doors with emphasis on mountain climbing. The manifestation was found to be a derivative of necrophilic fantasies, which fantasies served as a defense against phobic reactions to oneness with, and also separation from, the mother. The love of the "dead" mother and the need to master the fears of her, became the love and mastery of, or triumph over, the petrified dead aspects of mother nature. This derivative complex was felt as an experience of birth or as a wish for a rebirth.

---

[1]M. Bergmann. Personal communication.

The syndrome under consideration is homosexuality in the form of fantasies and acts. The primary identification is with the phallus of the phallic mother, though evidences of the prior breast identity are also present. The transformation wished for—to be separated from this mother and yet retain her image as an active, libidinized total self rather than that of the passive, castrated destructive one—was attempted unconsciously through the medium of homosexual fantasies and acts. This transformation was felt as a rebirth.

The rebirth fantasy is by no means confined to homosexuality or even the other syndromes mentioned above. Nevertheless, it is especially important in homosexuality because homosexuality is prominent in the other syndromes and because it appears to have a more central place in the multiple causes of homosexuality.

Freud (1905, 1920b, 1922) regarded homosexuality as the manifest expression of an attempt by the subject to compromise his own latent bisexuality by projecting it on the love object. Nunberg (1938a) believed that likewise the aim of the homosexual represents a compromise between aggressive and libidinal impulses. While both points of view are concerned with instinctual conflicts within the subject, the one with bisexuality and the other with cathexis, explicit in both is the idea of the wish for transformation through some form of integration. It appears to us that the rebirth fantasy represents at least one of its *modi operandi*.

The orientation of this study is the structural one and deals with the elements within the ego constellation and their cathexes. The fixation in the libido-ego development is believed to be at a point when the ego is emerging as a separate psychic structure and is engaged in the double tasks of integrating active and passive strivings and fusing libidinal and aggressive impulses. Identification is the field as well as the process of this double integration. Its final stage, assimilation, is not attained when the elements within the ego constellation are not miscible owing to the fact that together the passive incorporative aims and aggressive or destructive cathexes of the part-self images and of part-objects spell mutual annihilation. Homosexual acts and fantasies emerge in consequence.

This situation is the type referred to by Anna Freud (1936, p. 24) where "there is little opportunity for endopsychical displacement," or intrapsychic change, and the consequence is allopsychic displacement or acting out. Thus the homosexual perversion is at once an aborted identification and an acting out. No psychic change or real integration has taken place; merely a temporary reduction of psychic tension by externalization or projection of one or several of its ego fragments which are not miscible with the rest.[2] This compromise follows essentially the process of symptom formation as seen in the transference neuroses and is in accord with the principle of the repetition compulsion, derivative of the aggressive drive.

However, besides the tension-relieving aim, which is the more immediate and perhaps the more fundamental, homosexuality subserves another aim. It is that based on the significant need for restitution. Although both aims may be mediated by the rebirth fantasy, the restitutive aim appears to find a more complete expression in it. From this point of view the passive wishes in the homosexual (which seem to us to be the more basic ones), apart from being ends in themselves, aim at a change whereby appropriate and effective libidinal and constructively aggressive cathexes will be induced by love objects. This cathectic reconstellation is felt, visualized, or associated to as a rebirth. Thus, the psychological process of growth through identification, when aborted, chooses, instead, regressive processes of externalization or breaking away. These are the means employed in dissolving the psychological mother-child symbiosis, its prototype being the biological pattern of physical birth. Thus, processes of psychological growth come to be felt as experiences of birth—in effect, rebirth.

The restitutive aim is teleological and normative, albeit also ineffectual. The reason is that the acting out again uses passive and magical wishes as means to regain the goal of integration which the acting-out rendered impossible in the first instance. The restitutive aim is subserved by libido operating through the synthetic function of the ego (Nunberg, 1938a). It thus resembles the epinosic gain in the transference neuroses. In the latter, a weak ego attempts to salvage some small gains resulting from its weakness and capitula-

---

[2]This fact has also been recognized by Bychowski (1945) whose "ego introjects" seem to be larger aggregates stemming from later phases of development.

tion to the greater force of the id and superego. Here, however, restitution has a broader aim—promoting the further development, or synthesis, of the ego organization itself. The resemblance should therefore not obscure the far greater significance of the restitutive goal.

The case material is based on a study of a number of bisexual patients—pure or obligatory homosexuals rarely coming for treatment for the disorder as such—and exemplified in two clinical fragments. In the first patient, homosexual fantasies were common but acts were very rare. Both manifestations were seen *in statu nascendi* in relation to dissolution of paranoid projections. The second patient manifested only occasional strong, though fleeting, homosexual attractions.

Case A

The patient was a young man whose treatment extended over his entire adolescence and beyond. Beginning with school difficulties at 13, he developed ideas of reference and auditory hallucinations in which he was ridiculed, along with outbursts of aggressive behavior directed mostly toward his mother and neighbors. In a neighborhood marshland, he later channeled his destructive behavior on small animals—birds, cats, and rabbits, including mothers and their young ones. The bouts of destructiveness followed fantasies of nursing from his mother and becoming like her, desires for revenge on her, also being very annoyed with himself for wanting so strongly to be a baby. He devoted most of his working hours and time in treatment to an unending stream of passive fantasies about everyone he met. He felt he was a walking empty breast and wished to be filled up through all his apertures and sensory organs by the corresponding active organs. Later in treatment, the active breast became the active phallus. His mother was the model active person. He equated her verbal stream with the milk from her breast, and the latter with her phallus, which he visualized as a nipplelike extension of an intra-abdominal breast. This nipplelike genital organ would enter his penis in intercourse, flatten it out, and fill him with milk. He would then have the appearance of a little girl as a miniature form of his mother.

In the course of treatment he recognized that his ideas of

reference served as projections of his passive wishes and, to a lesser extent, of his aggression. When, after about two years, he recognized that he enjoyed talking to the analyst about his passive fantasies, he stopped talking about them and developed a sublimation for them. He studied and became a machinist, and for many months brought the products of his work to the analytic sessions and talked about them exclusively. He enjoyed being active and working with hard and heavy metal tools, using his strong muscles. He recognized in this the wish to change from having the hands of the little girl, the passive counterpart of mother, to a wish to be like the powerful mother. During periods when the work sublimation was not operative he thought everyone could see the little hands holding a large phallus instead of a machinist's tool. He found this so intolerable he had to leave his job. Considerably later he recognized a compulsion to belittle himself before his "audience." He expressed this as his need to convince people that he could not compete with them. He thus coupled regression from the oedipal conflict with masochism and paranoia.

With the recognition of his projections and their disappearance, latent passive anal and genital wishes in relation to all individuals became more prominent, but particularly in relation to men. At one point he allowed himself to be seduced at work by his foreman into participating in anal and sexual jokes and being "goosed." He admired the foreman for his abilities, the fact that he was a married man, also for his interest in teaching him and not fearing the patient's hostile wishes. The more he desired to identify with the foreman and the other men at work, the more he felt that he could not compete with them. For this he blamed his mother, and later his aunt, for belittling him in contrast to his father, uncle, and cousins. In time he recognized his competitiveness with his father in desiring to have his mother for himself. Any type of trained work meant to him chiefly competition with men. His inability to compete with any man accentuated all his passive wishes. But, in part, the passive fantasies were also motivated by a desire to become one with the admired, also hated, men in order to acquire some of their active strength. He expressed the wish to provoke a fight with one of the stronger men in order to get close and have some of his strength "rubbed off" onto him. He fantasied their eyes filled him up akin to nursing or that they were like cords which tied him to them. In moments of panic which would suddenly emerge in relation to "competition" when he did a good job—i.e., identified with the man he admired—he would be clearly aware of his need to escape into the safety of the nursling. He would imagine himself with the small hands of a little girl, his tools would drop out of his hands, he would leave his work and go home. Closeness to men heightened the wish to be active like them, but by the passive means of being tied to and penetrated by them as in the earlier fantasies in relation to his mother. The intensification of the passive wishes frightened him and made him feel guily. He warded off the fear and the guilt by means of paranoid projections. On several occasions the defense led to his resorting to the active role in fellatio with boys to strengthen the denial of his passive masochistic wishes even after that idea was projected.

During a subsequent phase in treatment he progressed to having sexual intercourse with women. Noting his preference for older women, he recognized his oedipal wishes toward his mother and particularly toward his aunt. He also vividly recalled his being seduced by the latter prior to the onset of his symptoms. He enjoyed the sexual act momentarily. But the largest elements in the enjoyment were sadistic and revengeful: the desire to triumph over the woman and degrade her. It was as if he could master the trauma of narcissistic hurts by a reversal; castrating the woman and himself becoming phallic. However, he was regularly disappointed. Upon separation from the sexual partner and awareness of his flaccid penis, he strongly felt that he took on her resemblance or that he was a miniature of her. He was angry at her and at the same time scornful of her and himself.

This aborted wish for a sudden magical transformation after the birth-rebirth pattern was disclosed in a fantasy during one of these postcoital reactive states. He visualized himself as "stuck" within the woman's body: the upper half inside and the lower outside, protruding and limp. The highly overdetermined and condensed meanings of this fantasy included oedipal wishes, as noted by himself; also the return to the mother to re-emerge phallic in the interchangeable images of phallic mother and/or phallic individuals—father, uncle, cousins. The aim was aborted by the postcoital separation. Separation was the forerunner and prototype of castration activated by seeing his small, flaccid penis. His partial success—the momentary castrated image of the female—helped further to strengthen his identical self-image, with the result that the trauma was activated rather than mastered by the sexual experience.

Case B

A 30-year-old married professional woman came for treatment because she was childless. Aware of strong, though fleeting, homosexual attractions, these frightened and depressed her. She would not act on them and even feared dwelling on the subject. She married a man she know was sterile but repressed the fact; it was obvious she married him because of this very fact.

From what she related and from what was worked out about her fears of the sexual life of a woman, and the consequences of its consummation upon her personality and symptoms, the following was significant. She was a happy child, felt she was an attractive little girl, played at house, etc. When she was 6 her mother went to work in her father's business and she felt deserted. Other early memories related to feeling she was an adopted child and being teasingly told by her mother that she was; also, that she was not as good as her older brother in taking the breast, necessitating early weaning. An outstandingly ecstatic early memory was of being taken into her mother's bed and held tightly with her back against the mother's abdomen. Because of additional factors, this memory was overdetermined and came to symbolize her phallic identification with (the phallic) mother, the undoing of separation anxieties, an escape from the dangers of femininity to herself and to mother, and the basis for her feeling attracted to women.

Behind the fears of sexuality were oral ideas of impregnation and sadistic ideas of abdominal birth. Numerous primal-scene anxieties included the probability of mother being dead whenever she found her asleep in the morning, and that mother began to die when she became pregnant with the patient. Her mother actually died from an abdominal malignancy when the patient was 14. Following this she developed amenorrhea and ideas that she was becoming masculine. Prior to this, for two years during prepuberty, she engaged in sexual play in what she described as mutual seduction with an uncle. This experience was both an acting out and a screen memory. It was a reaction to anxiety from primal-scene traumata, in which she shifted from her identification with the imperilled mother to that of the father-aggressor.

Later in her analysis she was able to characterize her illness as something abdominal. She now felt she was keeping her mother alive in her; this tied up with her feeling guilty that she was responsible for her mother's death. In another sense she also realized that she was herself partly dead—sick, depressed—where she was in contact with the avenging bad mother. To separate from her meant that one or the other might die, as if there were one life between them. The sickness was at times also experienced as an encapsulated phallus.

Sexual life as a woman meant for her to meet mother's fate. Pregnancy meant the same. She was unable to compromise her ambivalence toward her mother, which affected mother's phallic and feminine images. She felt left by mother during the pregenital phase of her life (early weaning and ideas of being adopted), but especially during the two phases of her oedipal development.

With the death of her mother, her father also left her. He broke up the family and became very dependent on a succession of women. He thus accentuated his weakness and his inadequate capacity to love his daughter and reciprocate her love. In this way he did not help to neutralize or compensate for the factors in the mother-child relationship which prompted her regression to the phallic self-image.

The determinants for both the homosexual attraction and the fear-avoidance of pregnancy were identical and may be listed summarily as follows: regression from the oedipal conflict; the good phallic mother was also a bad weaning mother; a wish to return to the blissful state of phallic oneness wherein mother transforms her into a phallic being and/or gives her a baby; finally the equation: separation=castration=giving birth=death.

During the final phase of the analysis the patient decided upon artificial insemination and conceived. During the first three months of her pregnancy, she refused to believe her obstetrician that she was really pregnant. At first she experienced many anxieties and calamitous expectations, then settled for a time on the idea of pseudociesis. At this time she had a dream in which she gave birth to two little boys. There was something unpleasant too: she tried to close a convertible and had a difficult time doing it. To the birth she associated a story about a polite lady who wished to have two boys. When she died at 90, they found in her abdomen two little old men, each of whom kept repeating to the other, "After you, my dear." She, too, wanted to have twins and then be done with that part of the life of a woman which caused her so much anxiety. The convertible meant to her folding or closing up below and reversion to the former state. The two little men stood for two penises or two testicles. She would avoid her mother's fate, repeating her fearscme ideas about mother's sexual life. She felt she was too sexual and had an image of herself as a beast; half man and half animal, fiercely sexual. She wished she was sexually traumatized like so many other children who are attacked and could then run and tell mother. The fear of death in identification with mother's fate was exchanged for the guilt of being identified with the sexually aggressive male. Also, she now wished to be freed from her identification with the male aggressor. The deepest wish in the dream represented an escape from the fearsome role of the adult female and the fiercely sexual role of the male into the image of the infantile fantasy of the phallic mother with all its benign and magical attributes. Similarly, homosexual attractions experienced as being drawn to breast-phallic zones represent wishes to be "converted" or reborn in the image of the phallic mother.

To sum up: Important determinants in homosexuality include fixation in the pleasure-ego phase of development, wherein the image of the self in the form of a phallus represents a part-object identity with the phallic mother; cathexes of the self-image mainly with destructive aggression, and a similar feeling about the cathexis of the object interferes with the process of identification. Homosexuality is a substitute process, an acting out, and serves purposes of relieving intropsychic tension and of restitutive wishes. In this paper, the latter are highlighted.

Chapter 11

On the Meaning of Agoraphilia*

Agoraphilia

Definition: *A fascination for the out-of-doors, viewing ruins, tramping on rock, climbing mountains to an inordinate degree, or to the extent of a hobby, sport, preferred type of vacation, or obsessive fantasies—all these phenomena are designated as agoraphilia.*

Example: *A patient described a very elated feeling he experienced in tramping in the open country, viewing large vistas and old ruins. He enjoyed the solid comfort of being supported while standing on rocks. He revelled in movement, in the free and deep respiration, in the spaciousness—all this especially while climbing mountains. The latter became his favorite vacation activity in which he indulged whenever possible.*

Related concepts: *Related to this concept are necrophilic fantasies of identification with and freedom from a dead person.*

In the course of delving into the etiologic roots of the stuttering syndrome, and other oral-narcissistic syndromes to which it always led, I was impressed by the central importance of the psychological symbiosis between mother and child and especially by the many

---

*Originally published in the *Journal of the American Psychoanalytic Association*, 1955, 3:701–709.

consequences of its incomplete dissolution. The point of fixation to which regression occurs later on is an early stage of ego organization. It is approximately that which has been variously designated: "pleasure ego" by Freud (1911a), "mouth ego" by Hoffer (1949), "part-ego" by Lewin.* Glover (1949) states that it is a period when the development of speech leads to the organization of the preconscious layers of the mind. The functioning of this early evolving ego state of the child, with its boundaries indistinct and still confluent with the mother, is by means of a sense of identity with her omnipotent total self or with parts of her body, especially breast or fantasied phallus. This functioning is archaic and pre-oedipal and has to be distinguished from the later true identifications emerging after resolution of the oedipus complex and even from their precursors which Freud called "primary identification" (1923). The distinction between the primitive and genuine identification is that the former strives to retain an archaic identity while the latter signifies a wish to assume, in the future, a new role—that of a love object; also, that in the former we are often dealing with an identity with a part-object while in the latter with an assumption of roles of a total object; finally, that the former state is beset with ambivalent cathexes while the latter strives to be unambivalent.

These remarks are germane because this paper is about one aspect of the incomplete dissolution of the primitive identification. Some other, and broader consequences of the same fixation I described in two recent papers. By way of introducing this one, I will merely state the findings of the first two: In the first paper, I traced certain determinants and deterrents in the study and practice of medicine to a wish to break with the primitive identification. The medical analysand regarded his typical patient as the mother and the typical therapeutic procedure as an ablation of the breast with which organ he was identified. This break was experienced as a kind of birth or rebirth, often accompanied by separation anxieties and agoraphobic reactions; on the other hand, the reactions to the sense of oneness with the mother were claustrophobic. In the second paper, the primitive identification was with the phallus of the phallic mother. The transformation wished for—to remain in

---

*B. D. Lewin. Personal Communication.

the image of the active, libidinized, ideal mother and yet be separated from her—was attempted unconsciously through the medium of homosexual fantasies and acts. This transformation was also felt as a rebirth.

In both studies separation fantasies were experienced in terms of a self-image, or self-representation, the designation used by Hartmann (1950) and Jacobson (1953), in the form of a castrated organ, cathected predominantly with aggressive energy and having the passive aims of reincorporation.

Out of the broad psychodynamic considerations of the two papers, from which the present is a fragment, the following are relevant here. The clinging between mother and child was generally attributed by the patient to the mother who was regarded as devouring and "bad"; the "good" mother, on the other hand, was the one who allowed separation. Conflicts arose from this danger of separation to both mother and child. The responsibility and guilt for initiating and effecting the separation fell on the child, who apparently survived at the expense of the mother. Thus, the mother was felt to have been sacrificed. Out of these conflicts and the attempts to solve them emerged the phenomenon of necrophilia, in which the mother, loved and feared as the corpse, was first introjected and then ejected.

These findings were corroborated by Brill's (1941) (See Ch. 9, p. 199) comprehensive study of this subject. According to him, the basic phenomenology of necrophilia includes a strong mother or grandmother fixation; fear of her death and the overcoming of that fear; aims of intercourse and mutilation of breast or body; vulturism; an inordinate craving for dermal contact; and sadomasochism. Similar findings are described in a paper entitled "A Necrophilic Phantasy" by H. Segal (1953). The patient's fantasy signified that he emptied his mother of all life and she became the corpse; this corpse he introjected and identified with himself and then projected.

Thus we have the following sequence: The first link consists of anxieties resulting from identity with mother and from separation from her leading to claustrophobic and agoraphobic reactions, respectively. The second link represents a counterphobic defense by means of necrophilia. The third link, which is the subject of this paper, is a derivative of necrophilia. The love of the "dead" mother and the need to master the fears of her become the love and mastery of, or triumph over, the petrified dead aspects of mother nature. We term this phenomenon agoraphilia and place it within the context of a wish for a symbolic birth or rebirth. A fascination for the out-of-doors, viewing ruins, tramping on rocks, climbing mountains to an inordinate degree, or to the extent of a hobby, sport, preferred type of vacation, or obsessive fantasies—all these phenomena are here designated as agoraphilia.

Discussion of the nature of this necrophilia derivative and its classification will be taken up after presenting the case material. The clinical examples which follow have been trimmed of all but the most essential facts.

Case A

A 20-year-old college student came for analysis because he was depressed, anxious, confused, and unable to continue with his studies. He was preparing to follow his father's profession. He regarded his father as weak and unsuccessful, which was contrary to fact, so impressed was he with his mother's more active and overbearing manner. Though both parents wished him to take the course, he became sick at school because he felt imprisoned by the maternal tie. He felt that his studies stretched endlessly in time, and he became anxious of what Lewin (1952) has referred to as "Mother Immortality." The imagery he used was both material and claustrophobic: he was wading through a fearfully long stretch of water, the other end of which he could not see.

The theme of being trapped and searching for release was often and variously repeated. Thus, in having a sexual relationship, it was necessary that he actually move into the woman's room, though this was followed by a series of physical and emotional withdrawals.

His many primal-scene fantasies included a dark enclosure, a flooring of liquid or semisolid consistency like mud, quicksilver, or seaweed which seemed to engulf him. Similar danger also threatened from a snake that had the bisexual characteristics of engulfing and attacking. Another series of fantasies contained sadistic and necrophilic elements. These included various forms of medieval torture, the most typical of which were directed against the female breast by means of needles being stuck into it, or by cruel pulling to effect ablation. That he himself was identified with the breast in this process was suggested by his occasional lifting his shirt away from his chest and saying that his nipples were sensitive. This was further expressed by his rapid flow of monotonous speech, which he enjoyed and which he "fed" for the entertainment, sleep-producing, and killing effect on the analyst. This was evidenced by the rapid succession of states of ecstasy, anxiety, and sleepiness, when he would sometimes turn and ask, "Are you there?"

In the following two fantasies, agoraphobic and claustrophobic elements are combined with those of necrophilia. In the first, he feels as if he were a small electric toy gadget. It is dead when disconnected and comes to life only when plugged into the socket in the wall. The idea is that there is one life in the primary identification which is interrupted in the separation and revived in the reunion. The same idea is repeated in the fantasy that he is like the Thief of Bagdad, who craves to steal into the palace. Once within it, he is trapped and remains in a sleep or deathlike state.

When these two fantasies were being worked through with him, he was asked whether he actually suffered from fears of closed spaces. He replied: "No, I have no claustrophobia; but I have an agoraphilia." Sophisticated in psychological terminology, he coined the latter term spontaneously. He described a very elated feeling he experienced in tramping in the open country, viewing large vistas and old ruins. He enjoyed the solid comfort of being supported while standing on rocks. He reveled in movement, in the free and deep respiration, in the spaciousness—all this especially while climbing mountains. The latter became his favorite vacation activity in which he indulged whenever possible. He had an awareness that mountains suggested breasts to him. Later, he became conscious that his fear of being as one with with his mother's breast led to his counterphobic, i.e., sadistic and necrophilic fantasies. These in turn were transformed into various aspects of "Mother Nature" in the inanimate form. This transformed mother was unambivalent. She did not cling and devour; she provided separation, gave firm support and enjoyable freedom of motion.

A follow-up interview six months after termination of analysis revealed two noteworthy facts. First, after working in another profession for three years, he suddenly and actively resumed his original professional studies, thus proving that he had mastered his fears of identification with his father. Obviously, one basis for the change was his break from the primitive identification with his mother. Second, the break was interestingly documented by a change in his appearance. For no other conscious reason than that he wanted to look different, he dieted, though he was not stout, and lost fifteen pounds. His trimmer look did make him appear different, and he said he felt happier with it. It was obviously the result of a wish for a new body image, after an experience which seemed to him, consciously and preconsciously, as a rebirth.

Case B

Outstanding in the life of J., a middle-aged single woman, was her harshly disciplined upbringing by a cold and controlling mother, abetted by a clinging, lonely maiden aunt who was also under the influence of her mother. This involvement lasted far into her adult life. Strong ambivalent attachments to women in authoritative positions disturbed her studies and her professional activities. The general pattern consisted of building up a *cause célèbre* based on complaints of belittlement. A wish to break away would be aroused early in the relationship, coupled with an inability to do so. Men friends were treated in a very similar manner.

Some time after Miss J.'s mother suffered a heart attack, Miss J. began to diet. Her aim was to reduce the size of her rather large breasts. The dieting at this time stood for an attempt to change her body image to one more appropriate, both realistically and symbolically. In the latter sense it meant shedding her breasts which represented the mother of whom she felt to be a part. This was expressed in a dream in which the bodice of her bathing suit was torn while she was swimming. The dream utilized an actual experience to express the symbolic wish.

While involved with these preoccupations, she took her mother on a visit to relatives who lived not far from the Canadian Rockies. She had visited there before, but this time she was possessed of a strong fascination and compulsion to climb one of the highest peaks in this region. She was especially enthusiastic about the idea of staying overnight at one point on the mountain and completing the climb and descent the next day. She stressed, in this connection, the thrill of emerging from the darkness of the night into the daylight on the mountain and completing the climb and descent the next day. She was certain that some debris at the base of this mountain represented lava which had erupted from it quite a long time ago. The lava was something born from the entrails of the mountain; it was also a token of a dangerous experience. She noted that a mountain opposite had the shape of a breast. She further stressed her fascination with the idea of the high stakes involved. The climb represented mastery of a critical danger, tested the endurance, and established the strength and freedom of movement of her limbs. Finally there was the pleasure of breathing in the rarefied air.

It is not difficult to recognize in this obsessive enthusiasm the idea of separation from the mother and rebirth in the form of a new body image, that is, alive and mobile. This reaction was stimulated by the fear of the mother's death, the need to separate from the primary identification, to master the fear of dying with her, and to act out the ecstatic possibility of the emergence of the self in a new body image. Here, too, we see the attempt to effect separation and master the fear of death by means of a necrophilic fantasy— projected onto the love of and triumph over "Mother Nature" in the petrified form of a mountain.

Discussion

Earlier, I stated my belief that agoraphilia is a derivative of necrophilia. However, before discussing its nature or classification, it may be noted here, on the basis of clinical and theoretical considerations, that agoraphilia appears not to be a derivative of, or reaction to, agoraphobia. Clinically, neither patient gave any history or current evidence of the latter. Both were able to leave home early and stay away for long periods. The first patient even ran away from home at about seven years of age. Furthermore, as a small boy, he invented a game, suggestive of what has been said regarding his primal-scene ideas about floors and footings, wherein he was able to circle or cross a room by stepping on different objects in it in lieu of touching the floor. Theoretically, according to Anny Katan

(1951, p. 50), "What is being displaced in agoraphobia is not the instinctual desire, but the product of defense. Incestuous anxiety is replaced by agoraphobia." Incestuous anxiety is not the central problem of the patients presented here, at least not as far as the syndrome under consideration is concerned. The problem is the final dissolution of the primary identification with the mother. Necrophilic fantasies and acts have a similar aim. How this aim is inadequately served by such means was pointedly illustrated by an adjunctive device invented by one of Brill's (1941) patients. He would indulge in a practical joke whereby he would induce his victim to enter a room in which there was a coffin. When the "corpse" was gazed upon, the patient who impersonated it would suddenly sit up in the coffin. The merriment of the perpetrator of the joke was in proportion to the fright of the onlooker. Obviously, the psychic economy of this joke consists of the exchange of the dread of identity with the dead for merriment associated with liberation from such an identity. The liberation may be experienced as a rebirth. Stated otherwise, the aim of this symptomatic act is to change the ambivalent (loved and feared) identity into an unambivalent or true identification which, as is well known, eliminates for practical purposes the aggression toward the object and results in a libidinized sense of similarity. Thus, what is hinted at in this symptomatic act—the need for a further step beyond the state encompassed by the necrophilic fantasy—is attained by the agoraphilia as defined in this paper.

What is the nature and classification of this attainment? In the first place, it is a derivative of a perversion or a perverse fantasy. As the latter stems from separation anxiety, its aim is counterphobic. In the end, however, the necrophilic remedy itself produces the opposite fear—that of being swallowed up or annihilated by the mother, who is experienced as an aggressively cathected, larger part-self. The countermeasure—rebirth through agoraphilia or rebirth and agoraphilia—is therefore also counterphobic. In the second place, then, it is an extended counterphobic structure. The combined positive elements in the two counterphobic reactions serve the defenses mentioned by Fenichel (1939): transformation of passive into active aims; identification with an object that frees rather than binds; contradiction of the possibility of castration; flight into reality. Rebirth through agoraphilia is then a special instance of flight into reality.

Finally, can we classify agoraphilia as a sublimation wherein "the impulse is channelized" (Fenichel, 1945), or as a reaction formation (the less frequent type) wherein "doing the same thing one originally feared serves the purpose of holding the original intensive wish in check" (p. 152)? The question may be answered if we extend the concepts of sublimation and reaction formation, used, as far as I know, to designate vicissitudes in id impulses exclusively, to transmutations in ego states. In that event, we may say that it depends upon the ego state. If the agoraphilia, symbolic of breaking the primitive identification, is enjoyed at a time when that break is still far in the future, we may say that we are dealing with a reaction formation. But if the break has been or is being accomplished, the agoraphilia represents a facilitation, or a celebration, of the event, and is therefore in the nature of a sublimation. In the first patient the agoraphilia was of long standing and prior to any change in the primitive identification. It was therefore largely a reaction formation, only latterly it was being transformed into a sublimation. In the second patient the agoraphilia emerged as a facilitation in the process of breaking of the primary identification precipitated by reality events. It may therefore be regarded as a sublimation.

Chapter 12

Federn's Annotation of Freud's Theory on Anxiety*

During the last few years of his life Federn conducted a seminar on Freud's works. While almost the entire time was devoted to the exposition of Freud's ideas, Federn would on occasion refer to and explain some of his own observations and concepts of ego psychology. The last book discussed was *The Problem of Anxiety* (Freud, 1926) as it is called in the Bunker translation (1936). Federn left me this book. In its margins he wrote a liberal number of annotations,[1] presumably when he was reviewing the material in preparation for the seminar. It seemed a fitting way to honor the memory of Federn on the occasion of the tenth anniversary of his death to present herewith these distinctive and challenging marginalia.

Many annotations are quoted in full, some are summarized. The organization of the material falls naturally into two related domains: Federn's distinctive views on the nature and functioning of the ego, on the one hand, and those on anxiety, on the other.[2] For the sake of greater clarity I decided to include only the marginalia dealing with these subjects insofar as they are interrelated. Fortunately, these constitute the largest number.[3]

---

*Originally published in the *Journal of the American Psychoanalytic Association*, 1963, 11:84–96.

[1]The entire body of annotations, running into twenty typewritten pages, has been placed in the Brill Library of the New York Psychoanalytic Society. Federn wrote these annotations in English.

[2]For a description of Federn's psychology of the ego, the reader is referred to Bergmann (1963)—Ed.

[3]Those omitted touch on the problem of the choice of neurosis or health-reaction types, types of resistance and defense, and variations in affect.

Federn's final annotation is written in bold hand, and it epitomizes the spirit in which all the comments are made:

> Whoever shall take the pain of deciphering, shall be aware of my reluctance against changing or adding anything to Freud's presentations. I did it with deepest awe for his discoveries in the field of mental processes, and even more of the depth of the unconscious. Whenever I proceeded farther, I followed and did not leave behind his paths. I go with—not against—him. I had to do it because of my greater and better knowledge of the ego-psychology.

Divergences Regarding Development and Meaning of Anxiety

To place Federn's comments in sharp focus it is necessary to start with Freud's theses about anxiety and his argument for changing from the first to the second theory of anxiety. I shall point up those nodal links in Freud's chain of thoughts to which Federn's marginalia relate. First, the change in the theory of anxiety involved only its third category—neurotic anxiety—and not real or actual anxiety. The bridge between the two classifications was the concentration of instinctual tension in anxiety. To this, two elements were now added: (1) that concentration was regarded as traumatic, i.e., its essence was economic—a painful flooding by instinctual energy of portions of the psychic and physical apparatus; (2) the historical factor; this flooding repeated an earlier experience, the birth experience, which became the prototype for later traumatic experiences. Aspects of the neonate's behavior were further linked with the hysteric's similar physical manifestations. In both, the early anxiety was deemed purposive and efficient; the later-developing anxiety, without purpose and inefficient. Closer observation, especially of the phobic anxiety of Little Hans and the Wolf Man, led Freud to believe that anxiety is more often purposive than otherwise. The next step related the purpose with the external danger situation and its concomitant internal traumatic situation whence stemmed anxiety as a signal, i.e., a signal for defense. Thus, there is transformation from automatic traumatic anxiety in a causal sequence to that of signal anxiety as a teleological phenomenon. The stages consisted of early purposive anxiety, later useless anxiety, and still later anxiety which may often become useful. The search for the etiology of the external danger which in turn produces the internal traumatic situation focused on the phenomenon of separation in its classical phases of weaning, training, loss of maternal love, and loss of superego love. Finally, the second anxiety theory changed the role played by repression from that of primary trigger of anxiety to that of secondary reaction to anxiety.

Freud begins his critique of his first theory of anxiety by an attempt to answer what he called the riddle of how repression can turn pleasure into unpleasure. He states (pp. 17–18)[4] that the riddle of "transformation of affect in repression disappears when we consider that as a result of repression, the excitation arising in the id altogether fails to discharge." He makes the power of the ego responsible for repression and then proceeds to relate, ". . . the way in which this surprising manifestation of power becomes possible to the ego." The following two elements are involved here: (1) the ego's capacity to transform one affect into another—pleasure into unpleasure, and an instinct into an affect—libido into anxiety; and (2) the strength of the ego vis-à-vis the id and the manifestation of that strength through the mechanism of repression.

Federn's view varied in a number of ways regarding both elements just mentioned. As to transformation of affect, Federn wrote, "This problem does not exist. The impossibility of urge-satisfaction is felt as severe unpleasure which creates repression. It is also possible that by will power, the ego—in some people—inhibits the biological, and as a consequence the psychological, discharge of the content of the id. Yet, in most cases it is enough to dislike, or repulse satisfaction, that unpleasure develops. . . ."

However, apart from the idea of transformation of libido into anxiety, Federn was keenly aware, as was Freud, of the close relation and tie between libido and anxiety. Federn's annotations made several references to that relation. Thus, one of Federn's main tenets, which will be elaborated further, is that *anxiety flows directly from an inhibition of flight* from a feared object. The inhibition in turn is caused by ambivalence—the libidinal masochistic tie to the same object; hence, the connection between libido and anxiety. Another example of their agreement on the close connection between libido

---

[4]All quotations are from the Bunker translation of 1936—Ed.

and anxiety is stated by Federn as follows: "Any intensification of the quantity, or change of quality, of libidinal needs and tensions—also true for the aggressive cathexis—produces an activation of earlier unsatisfied urges, with the emergence of painful and pleasurable affects, and produces, in other words, an affectively more labile state." Elsewhere, Federn states that, "whereas actual libidinal experience diminishes or even counteracts anxiety, which is due to real feared objects, it does increase the neurotic anxiety. In the latter case, the quality of danger remains whether the libidinal impulse is inhibited by conscious fear or by repression operating unconsciously." At one point Federn calls the creation of anxiety accompanying the blocking of the free discharge of libido "the physiopsychologic parallel." Thus, while he recognized the validity of the phenomena of the "actual" neuroses, he did not isolate them from the psychodynamics applicable to the psychoneurosis.

Federn's acceptance of Freud's new concept that the ego's anxiety produces repression is in the generic sense of the ego's involvement with anxiety, but he asserts his belief that anxiety is almost always experienced in an automatic, i.e., passive, way. "The ego is the primal site of origin of repression rather than originator of it. The passive reaction of the ego, flight, is being hindered by a libidinal attachment to the dangerous object, and it is notably this aggravation which gives rise to anxiety on the part of the ego." According to Federn, "even though the ego in anxiety reacts with hallucinatory strength, it does so in response to present causes and those linked to the past," but he emphasized that "the reaction is automatic and passive." In contrast, Freud treats neurotic anxiety almost always as the opposite of something that is automatically and causally determined; he sees it as something motivated by a purpose or design, that is to say, he has a teleological view. Freud uses the analogy of a vaccine having the aim of mobilizing the defensive forces.

I shall next consider the sequence of events producing anxiety according to Federn. Because the annotations here are somewhat elaborate, I present only those which deal with the nub of the subject. Freud regarded the factor of separation, in its various manifestations, as the key danger situation. Here, Federn's note reads: "Freud's equations—separation equals danger; anxiety equals signal of danger, are a semantic error. Separation itself does not create anxiety, but the *conditions* of the separating process which include the consequences of awareness of helplessness and the dread of the object." Freud believed that it is the state of helplessness which explains the traumatic nature of a danger situation. According to Federn, "it is the ensuing feeling of paralysis from terror which constitutes the traumatic nature of a danger situation." Federn now details the sequence of events more specifically as follows:

> The ego faces danger and feels either courage or rage, or the readiness to fight. If the urge to fight is stopped, the emotion of dread follows. Then the ego senses or remembers its weakness and flees. Then, when the flight is hindered, a feeling of terror results—it is a feeling of nearness to death. Full anxiety is hallucinated terror; a signal is an approach to danger, and signal anxiety is hallucinated danger. The hallucinated danger is a means of defense against terror. In other words, signal anxiety is a defense against real anxiety. In signal anxiety only the ego boundary is cathected; in real anxiety, the whole ego. The same relation holds for a signal of dread and real dread. The anxiety signal (not the complete anxiety) is a later phobic mechanism, but does not belong to "actual" anxiety and not to symptom formation.

It may be relevant to recall here that, as mentioned above, Freud first formulated the concept of signal anxiety on the basis of his two examples of phobic anxiety.

In several annotations Federn maintains that an "affect is much more than a symbol; it is an experience of an ego boundary of a typical nature." He states, "anxiety primarily does not have a function; it is evidence of damage and of a functional defect." And he repeats that it is the hindered flight that is the nuclear cause of anxiety. Finally, according to Federn,

> ... the physiologic discharge processes and the historic repetitive nature of anxiety are not sufficient in themselves for its understanding without the assumption of mortido, i.e., feelings of terror or nearness of death on the one hand, and on the other, the libidinal pull toward it—the (instinctual and affective) ambivalence or the masochism which inhibits flight. ... Anxiety, because of the hindered flight also contains in it libidinal components—an inversion of the normal instinctual circulation. ... After unsuccessful repression, anxiety remains as a desire for hindered flight. Without ambivalence, it is possible no new anxiety would develop after unsuccessful repression.

The Role of the Ego

It seems clear that the different views on anxiety derive from different conceptions of the nature and role of the ego in psychic life. I start with Freud's presentation of aspects of the ego and follow with Federn's comments. Freud introduces the subject with the remark (p. 24) that the ego has separated itself from the id in that it has become its differentiated and organized portion, yet it is identical with it. In 1923 (pp. 57–58) he described the ego's impotence and apprehensiveness toward the id and the superego; in 1926, on the other hand, he contends (pp. 24–26) that the ego has the power of control in admitting component elements of the id into consciousness and external behavior, and that in repression it is in control at both places. He explains the discrepancy in strength on the basis that junction or oneness of the separated portion with the energies of the id and superego spells strength, but that its disjunction, tension, or conflict with these energies makes its weakness apparent. Furthermore, an element of ego strength in repression is that the ego is an organization. Another aspect of ego strength is evidenced in its function of synthesis, whereby it uses desexualized energy and is thus close to the id. Still another aspect is from the insight into its "modus operandi of repression." These factors are deemed by Freud to be adequate bases for assigning to the ego that purposive integrating potency which, among other affects, can create anxiety as a signal for defensive purposes.

Federn's marginal annotations contain many references to this strength aspect of the ego, and they are at variance with Freud's views. I will mention a few that are typical. In discussing phobias, Freud notes that "varied means are employed by the ego in its defense against the id." Instead of "means are employed," Federn writes "phenomena occur"—the more passive form. Further, when Freud refers to inhibition as the expression of a functional limitation of the ego, Federn states more explicitly that "the limitation is imposed on or starting from the ego." Again, when according to Freud the ego renounces functions so as not to have to undertake fresh efforts at repression and avoid conflict with the id, Federn's rejoinder is that "the ego's renouncing is because of its being hindered by the id and by the superego." In discussing phobias, Freud writes, "the ego is anxious on account of demands of the libido and the anxiety is the ego's motive and incentive for repression." Here, Federn substitutes "primal origin" for "motive." Finally, referring to Little Hans, Freud notes that his ego must intervene against the libido cathexis because of the danger of castration. Federn writes here, "it is more adequate to say the ego dreads object cathexis (i.e., flees from) rather than intervenes against object cathexis."

At one point, Freud summarizes some of the means employed by the ego such as turning aside the libido, impairment of execution of function, inhibition of social conditions, prevention by precautionary measures, discontinuance by development of anxiety, reaction of protest to the act and desire to undo it. Here, Federn offers his contribution, which is a classification consisting of three categories: "1) locality—ego cathexis; 2) decrease or increase of cathexis; 3) loss of libido or interference by mortido. This last could lead to loss of will power or inhibition and to depression as well as anxiety." Thus, Freud's summary contains descriptive and dynamic elements; Federn's classification is one of economic and energic factors, in other words, vicissitudes in ego cathexis.

After these examples of Federn's views, his comments on Freud's warning against the alleged excessive emphasis on the passivity of the ego are in order. Regarding the ego controls, Federn writes,

> This is inexact. The ego influences the entrance to a moderate degree by will power and attention, yet usually the ego boundary moves and changes in a passive way through urge (drive) representations and stimuli whose cathexis is increased by preconscious and unconscious changes. The ego can interfere with this and regulate the entrance by a "motor" inhibition, by an egotizing "trial" cathexis, by pulling "switches" which give place and way to associations in a desired direction and diminish the energy of associative choices in other directions—will power, attentiveness of an active nature, and interest are used by the ego—yet *mainly* attention, repression, and also regression are passive procedures.

Regarding the id-ego relation: Federn's comment on Freud's statement that the ego is a separated and a specially differentiated portion of the id, reads: "It is rather the reverse: the id is largely a series of repressed or 'lived out' ego states. The ego begins with the starting of life." The alleged weakness of the ego in a state of disjunction from the id is noted by Federn as "the giving way to instinctual urges, i.e., the ego becomes masochistic." He then identifies ego strength with "sadism and normal sexuality." Apropos of Freud's statement that the ego is an organization and the id is not (p. 24), Federn writes: "In Freud's opinion, the id is only a collective name but no unit." To this Federn adds that "while the ego is an organization built up out of unified feeling cathexis, as well as out of conscious perceptions, the id is an archaic and biological organization plus repressed ego states. The repressed does not get any assistance from other portions of the id. The repressed remains isolated, but joins part of the id." As to repression demonstrating the strength of the ego, Federn notes: "It is a false assumption that our 'ego' represses by its own action—yet repression itself is a passive experience of the ego's flight."

In a similar fashion Federn comments on what Freud called "the compulsion to synthesis (p. 26) within the ego—one which produces adaptation, a binding of the symptom to itself, and gives narcissistic gratification from the secondary gain of illness, etc. To Federn this compulsion to synthesis on the part of the ego is "nothing but the need to overcome ambivalence and the pain-pleasure principle, especially in relation to one interest overshadowing all others." Federn then underscores the following: "Superego, libido, will power, reason, are uniting and synthesizing forces of the ego. Yet the 'unified cathexis' is no synthesis, but the essence of the ego." To Federn, then, the idea that the ego is an organization has a different meaning. More than the functions of perception, repression, and synthesis, the ego is for him the core of the personality since birth and possesses continuous and coherent cathexes.

We glimpse here a sketchy outline of Federn's main contribution. Basic to his view of the ego is that, at its center,

> ... it is a phenomenon of psychic experience, an *Erlebnis* of unified, ongoing feelings of one's physical and mental self. Free-flowing, automatic, qualitative changes are characteristic of the ego boundary. The boundary is cathected with libido and may therefore choose what satisfies the libido. That may have the appearance of synthesis, but is not. The ego state is fixed, and it digests all actual experiences. The boundary is in contact with id, superego, and objects in the external world. As a result of guilt, for example, in compulsion neurosis especially, the plasticity or free-floating attention at the ego boundary

is changed into a more rigid state. Hence, our need to "educate" the compulsive neurotic to associate freely. To withdraw cathexis unity[5] essential to the go is really beyond our ability. One does not succeed in intentionally not thinking of something.

[Again elaborating somewhat on what was already mentioned . . .] what looks like synthesis when the ego boundaries change their contents is that a strong cathexis of one interest overshadows all others.

The sum total of cathectic energy, Federn believes, is made up of three basic urges—love, life, and death energies. (The distinction between love and life energy is not described.)

To Federn, regression and the unconscious operation of earlier ego states play an important role in psychopathology. For example, in speaking about working through, Freud justified its necessity, following the conscious recognition of resistance by the patient, because of the further need to overcome the resistance of "the ego's unconscious prototypes exerting their attraction upon the repressed instinctual process" (p. 105). Federn interpreted this as follows: to Freud, the ego's "unconscious prototypes" refer to the instinctual drives and their inertia in the id, and are synonymous with Freud's idea of the repetition principle which involves the id. "In that case," Federn concludes, "working through could not be of help." To him, what is responsible for the operation of the repetition principle are fixated early ego states and their strong resistances to being made conscious; working through means overcoming these. Thus to Federn, what is often referred to as

> . . . regression, affect, memory, symbol, or fascination for earlier libidinal patterns is but the reappearance of previously repressed ego states. . . . Affect is much more than a symbol. It is an experience at the ego boundary with instinctual cathexis which differs from that of the object representation. Thus, anxiety also may stem from the earliest levels of ego formation—phylo- and biogenetic—appearing not only as such but also as hunger from the pleasure experience of nursing. . . . One must extend Freud's second anxiety theory over all kinds of unpleasure.

---

[5] Concerning "cathexis unity," Weiss (1952, p. 8) says: "Federn describes the ego as an experience, as the sensation and knowledge of the individual of the lasting or recurrent continuity, in time, space, and causality, of his bodily and mental life. This continuity is felt and apprehended as a unity."

A final word on ego strength and weakness, according to Federn. Freud defines counter cathexis as an alteration of the ego when it assumes an attitude that is antithetical to an instinctual tendency which is to be repressed. Federn formulates it as "the discrepancy between the quality of cathexis of the object representation and that of the relevant ego boundary. It is this contrast which maintains repression; it is the manifestation of resistance. Intrinsically countercathexis represents ego strength. It may mean a readiness to cathect opposing, alternative, or substitutive functions, or a guarding against repressed complexes by opposition and fear. Another source of countercathexis is the repressed and therefore inaccessible ego states which resist reawakening. A third source is the object representations which are cathected with mortido, more especially when repressed." Regarding ego weakness Federn stresses two factors: "one, the pain-pleasure principle and its excessive premium, causing the ego to accept neurosis and suffering from symptoms as a lesser evil than the threat of castration in its varied forms; the other, which is related—the libidinal tie to feared objects—i.e., ambivalence and masochism which interfere with flight and produce anxiety."

Comments

It is hoped that the major annotations quoted here, representing illustrative fragments of Federn's ego psychology, will stimulate further interest in Federn's writings. Such a pursuit will, in my opinion, help to broaden the view of the ego beyond the current almost exclusive definition of it in terms of disparate functions only (Hartmann, 1950). Freud found that the ego has a physical base and a cathexis of its own; he visualized it as an organization, a major function of which is to synthesize its perceptions and activities. *A priori*, it seems more tenable that an organization which synthesizes functions is itself integrated and experienced as such. The fact is that, though the ego feeling is generally experienced preconsciously, it may with some effort be experienced consciously; and it is certainly clearly felt under special conditions of health and illness such as fatigue, hypnagogic and depersonalized states, and particularly in association with anxiety wherein it is not infrequently experienced in the form of blank hallucinations, distrubances in identity, etc.

It must be underscored here that Federn accepted the ego functions as a partial definition of the ego. He wrote about ego feelings not on an either-or basis but as something distinct and different. Disturbances in ego feelings, reflecting vicissitudes in ego cathexis, do produce various symptoms, including a severe form of anxiety. These symptoms may operate during and following states of conflict. The dynamics of these conflictual states cannot explain all of these symptoms, which must be understood as entities per se. Here Federn's contribution is noteworthy in that he called attention to the necessity to recognize more than defense in symptom formation. He stressed that some symptoms bespeak manifestations of ego breakdown, a fact not at all unique if we keep in mind Freud's teaching that in all symptoms some form of ego failure is implicit. When it is also explicit, it may often take the form of disturbances in ego feelings. While Federn does speak mainly of the sensory-affective state of the ego at its core and its boundaries and relatively less of specific functions of the ego, Freud deals almost entirely with the integrating and problem-solving functions of the ego.

What is the basis for the difference between the two? The question is complex and may be answered variously. Waelder puts this problem succinctly and gives his answer. He writes:

> It is legitimate to define the ego as an integrative, problem-solving agent; and equally legitimate to define it as the seat of sensations about oneself and the outside world. But one cannot do both at the same time without further investigation, i.e., one cannot take it for granted that integrative activities and sensations are always so closely associated that they must be attributed to the same agency. The ego of Federn, which experiences the boundary between the self and the outside world, or between different parts of the self, need not be the same as the ego of Freud which signals danger and represses dangerous impulses (1960, p. 187).

It seems to me, though both Freud and Federn deal with the same agency, the ego, they concentrate on different facets within it. However, they are at one in thinking of the ego not in health but as it is affected by psychopathology; for anxiety, whether purposeless or purposeful, is automatic and, as was well noted by Waelder (1929, p. 64), "the automaticity of anxiety defines neurosis in general." Freud stated, "The healthy individual masters his early traumatic and allied anxieties, becomes free of them, and has no further need to utilize them in any way. Why some individuals are capable of this mastery and not others is the nuclear determinant for neurosis" — a distinction Freud raises but does not answer. But in spite of Freud's and Federn's agreement on this fact, we can be reasonably certain that each had in mind types of patients who were not very close to each other within the wide range of psychopathology. When *Hemmung, Symptom und Angst* was written, Freud was again involved with the psychoneurosis, his earlier interest, while Federn progressively interested himself in the psychoses and allied narcissistic disorders.* Federn was thus impressed by the more pervasive passivity and masochism he encountered, while Freud noted the relatively more circumscribed and benign ego pathology in his material.

Additional Readings

1. A. A. Brill. Necrophilia. *Journal of Criminal Psychology*, 1941, 2:433–443; 3:51–73.

2. H. Segal. A necrophilic phantasy. *International Journal of Psycho-Analysis*, 1953, 34:98–102.

---

*Editor's Note: The reader may be interested in the following communication from Dr. Weiss concerning Federn's reactions to this book by Freud:

September 18, 1958

Dear Dr. Glauber:

I thank you very much for your letter. Dr. Federn has shown me that book of Freud "Hemmung, Symptom und Angst" with his note on the margins of the pages. He told me that Freud must have regretted having written that book or having expressed many ideas which that book contained.

To write a paper utilizing Federn's marginal annotations would be a worthwhile enterprise.

Mr. Ernst Federn wrote me about the place of the group to celebrate the anniversary of Federn's death in 1960 through a scientific meeting or some publications. I shall certainly participate. . . . I am writing now a book "The Ego and Its Worlds," meaning the interest and external worlds, beyond the ego boundaries, and will dedicate this book to the memory of Paul Federn. . . .

Very cordially,

[signed] Eduardo Weiss

Chapter 13

Dysautomatization: A Disorder of Preconscious Ego Functioning*

Dysautomatization

Definition: *Disturbances in such basic automatisms as breathing, speaking, locomotion, etc.*

Example: *Stuttering, asthma, tics, astasia-abasia.*

Related Concepts: *Related to this concept are the phenomenaa of the actual neurosis and disturbances in ego cathexis.*

Many, if not most, of the ego functions operate automatically, which is to say, preconsciously. It then follows that a disturbance affecting the automaticity, and with it the preconscious qualities of such functioning—which I refer to as a *dysautomatization*—is indeed a fundamental disturbance. This paper will consider certain phenomenologic and psychoanalytic aspects of the problem.

Some functions, like perception, though usually operating preconsciously, may under special circumstances of learning or defensive alertness take on more *quality*, the Freudian expression for increased cathexis, through focused attention, leading to

---

*Originally published in the *International Journal of Psycho-Analysis*, 1968, 49:89–99.

At the time of his death, in December, 1966, Dr. Glauber had completed this paper except for the summary, added by the editor, Helen M. Glauber, and Dr. H. Robert Blank. It was read by Dr. Peter Laderman at the May, 1967, meeting of the Westchester Psychoanalytic Society.

conscious cathexis of the functioning. This would be especially true for the monitoring or feedback component of this complex operation. We might call such functioning *facultative*, in contrast to another group of functions that are always in health obligatorily preconscious.

It is the clinical experience with the latter group, the so-called ego automatisms, more particularly the function of speech and its disturbances, that stimulated this paper and contributed to the major part of the clinical data and theory. Implications for other automatisms are suggested. In addition, disturbed fluency in muscular coordination and lability of optimal tonicity (hyper- and hypotonicity) are discussed. Characteristic of dysautomatization is a difficulty in the smooth transition from automatic to conscious functioning and an occasional combination of the two. An example of the latter is the clumsiness of some stutterers in shifting from extemporaneous speaking without notes to speaking from notes, or to reading, and vice versa.

While normally connections exist among the unconscious, preconscious, and conscious functioning, there are also normal barriers interspersed among them offering more or less difficulty in transition from one level to another. In the presence of dysautomatization, however, the balance between the three is disturbed. It is noteworthy that the attempt at their conscious control is in the nature of an inhibition. Inasmuch as the inhibition often serves as an adaptation (i.e., either as an inhibition of expression per se or as inhibition alongside an expression-symptom) it itself becomes secondarily automatized. This is evidenced clinically by the patient being not at all, or hardly, or only peripherally, aware of his jerky, iterative, or tonic speech.

One reason for this presentation is to exemplify a syndrome of much wider distribution than the example might suggest. Another reason is theoretical: to illustrative intra-ego conflicts (conscious vs. preconscious functioning) as between real or phenomenological rather than theoretical entities. So much for a sketchy overview of the disturbance of an automatism referred to here as dysautomatization; it will be discussed in more detail later on.

First, we must concern ourselves with the nature of the disorder. It can best be described as a developmental process, the process of acquisition of the ego function of speaking, and its deviation into a pathologic syndrome. This viewpoint emphasizes a unique fact that stuttering emerges while speech in its advanced form—the automatic form—is still in the process of being mastered. Speech, like other ego functions in their developments, commences as narcissistic play, then progresses by playful conscious imitation and unconscious identification toward utilitarian aims beyond play (meaningful verbalization) involving objects and object relations. In the process, the quality of cathexis changes from unconscious to conscious and preconscious. Finally, the process operates as an automatism, that is to say, that transformation from thoughts to words and the supervisory tasks of monitoring and feedback of sound and fluency take place preconsciously.

At moments of new learning experiences or of danger, situations which might be called potentially traumatic, some conscious, or even some total self-conscious, qualities or cathexes are added, resulting in some added efficiency or acquisition, though the burden of working with two monitors is evidenced by a lessening of fluency. However, in almost all cases the added attention cathexis and the shifting back into the regular automatic pattern are rapid and uneventful. The normal developmental pattern of the automatism, then, is: first, simple, smooth automatic expression of lalling and echolalia (unconscious, or id); then, less fluent, halting imitation (conscious, or conscious ego); finally, effortless, fluent, most efficient expression (preconscious, preconscious ego). The essence of the pathologic formation is the repetitive intrusion of some attempts at conscious monitoring in a process that has already developed to the more efficient phase of automatic functioning and that still persists in such functioning. In addition there are also intrusions of sounds from the earliest tension discharge or id level. Thus there is an alteration in the quality of preconscious cathexis (Kris, 1950), and its characteristic style of fluency is modified. Despite regressive intrusions, complete regression to a former modality does not occur. In addition, the new cathexis is not firm, but labile. The effect is shifting from hypercathexis to decathexis. What can produce such an effect? The answer is trauma.

In dealing with trauma in the context of its disturbing an

automatism, it is difficult to avoid a historical reference, although brief, to its place in the context of the neuroses. At the same time the comparison and the contrast between the two syndromes (dysautomatization and neurosis) are significant. Freud (and his followers) ceased referring to the traumatic theory of the neuroses when Freud discovered (1897–1902) that it was the fantasied trauma that was the nucleus of the neurotic disturbance. Later on, the term trauma was limited to its use in the traumatic neuroses, thought to function, paradoxically, "beyond the pleasure principle" (Freud, 1920a). Actually, both the psychoneuroses and the traumatic neuroses contain the strangulated affects stemming from blocked libidinal and aggressive drives. However, their ratios differ in the two neuroses, with the aggressive drives more directly involved in the traumatic. Certainly when we refer to the traumatic neuroses we have in mind real traumata, i.e., overwhelming stimuli from the environment. These as suggested by Greenacre (1952), may have an organizing effect on the fantasy and produce a state of shock which may also initiate a new psychic trauma. The tendency to repeat is present in both: in the psychoneurotic it takes the form of anticipatory signal anxiety; in the traumatic, the breakthrough in speech of elements of the original trauma with or without elements of defenses along with massive anxiety. On the other hand, the characteristic tendency to repeat in traumatic neuroses may be related to the well-known phenomenon of libidinization of elements of the traumatic experience or other elements associated with or immediately antecedent to them. The two syndromes contrast in the way anxiety is handled; the psychoneurotic develops a (new) defense against it in the form of a sensitized anticipation, which we call signal anxiety, to ward off anxiety mounting to a disorganizing degree. The traumatic-neurotic deals with it by total repression during wakefulness only to have the anxiety break through the weaker defenses of the sleep-ego. Repetitions are more episodic and dramatic, signal anxiety more consistent. But the two syndromes are comparable in that what are impaired are specific drive and affective manifestations, leading to fixations and difficulties in development, and impaired resolution of conflicts. The ego as such is only secondarily affected and then only or mainly in the circumscribed areas of the fixated drives and affects.

How does trauma affect an ego automatism like speech? Before this can be answered, we might first inquire into the nature of the trauma. Interestingly, there is often a sudden, sharp, real trauma, a minor accident such as a fall, or an injury, or an acute illness, which immediately precedes the onset and precipitates it. However, the determining trauma is the composite, earlier, long-range series of events of which the precipitating trauma is possibly a proof or a consequence. In the broadest terms, the essence of the trauma is the child's feeling of separation from the primary identification with the mother. This is an actual experience for the child—and undoubtedly it is later elaborated and organized by him—an uncanny intuitive awareness that suddenly, even though momentarily, the mother withdrew from him. She actually does so perhaps only in a recurrent fleeting moment of anxiety when her own much-wished-for state of symbiosis with the child is interrupted. That moment is generally one when the child shows some ego mastery, often of a slight degree, or any reminder of difference between them. She becomes aware of separateness, of "twosomeness," and almost imperceptibly moves from an unselfconscious, enjoyable involvement with the child, whether it is nursing or the teaching of words, to one of quizzical or anxious observation of him. The child instantly reflects this change and reacts similarly. We might describe it as a bit of flight, a bit of selfconsciousness. In metapsychologic terms, there is a cathectic shift from the play of object libido to one of narcissistic libido; more accurately, from attempts at object libido or completing self-differentiation to an earlier ego state—the ego-cosmic or the undifferentiated state. The mutually enjoyable game of teaching-learning words and speech is particularly vulnerable to such interruptions of and returns to the fluency and automaticity of the speech. In this type of pathogenic milieu, interruptions in such processes as nursing, walking, talking accompany many, if not most, of the stages of ego development and differentiation in the child.

Following from these experiences, processes of completing phases of ego development and moving on to new ones come to be regarded by the child as dangerous, not only to himself but to the mother as well. In the description that follows of the (more or less definitive) stages of this pathological development, we shall see how the fixation of one or several ego automatisms becomes organized in the mental life of the patient and affects his self-representation and total functioning.

The above is a sketchy fragment of an aspect of the mother-child relationship as it relates to the problem of some automatic functions. The anal and phallic-urethral meaning of this child to its mother and its connection with the phallic ideals of the mother and her forebears I have already described (see Ch. 4). Here, only the complex of trauma and its repercussions are being highlighted.

Something should be said about specificity in choice of symptom. It has been my observation from personal communications and from the literature that this problem is generally not considered in practice. There are gross lacunae in our knowledge about specificity. I have been impressed by (1) the ambivalence of the nursing mother—a "stuttering" type of nursing, impression ambivalence on the oral apparatus which is later borrowed for purposes of speech; (2) the peculiar sensitiveness to speech on the part of the mother who herself diagnoses stuttering in her child prematurely (during the normal early iterations), a sensitiveness partly related to the not infrequent stuttering of her father or brother to whom she related competitively or by idealization (the phallic-urethral exhibitionism has been mentioned); and (3) by the fact that this is a disturbance during the learning phase of an automatic function (or before it is fully learned) and that in a sense, as a result of trauma, it has been "learned" incorrectly and in large part has been secondarily automatized and experienced by the stutterer as his "normal" speech.

What remains now is to relate the effects of the trauma on the production of the symptom and the effect of both trauma and symptom on the total personality. Both symptom and total personality are unique in that they differ significantly from the classical psychoneurosis. In stressing this fact I am thinking of stuttering as a prototype for a large group of disorders to which the same pathologic formation of dysautomatization pertains, especially some disorders of perception, thinking, and learning.

Trauma and traumatic anxiety together can be described. It is a situation and state of being and feeling passively overwhelmed by stimuli from two foreign territories, the external world and the

inner unconscious world, both inundating or threatening to inundate the ego, which experiences a feeling of dissolution or nearness to death. Part of the feeling of helplessness and passivity is due to the libidinal masochistic ties to the feared object. The painfulness of the state is due to accumulated and undischarged instinctual tensions. The anxiety is due to cathectic charges within the ego in the nature of a defusion, whereby the libidinal energies become concentrated inwardly and the aggressive energies gravitate to the ego boundaries at the points of contact with the external world and the inner unconscious world. As a result of this drive splitting, the libidinal energies function passively while the aggressive energies function actively. This change is understandable and in line with the clinical observation that the defensive reaction to trauma is the shift to the active modality. An example is the defense reaction of identification with the aggressor (Anna Freud, 1936).

In many life situations, especially those of new learning or danger, a thrust toward activity in attention, perception, and performance may be highly desirable if not essential. This is not so, of course, when automatic processes like speech are involved which include complex muscular interactions. Here, automatic action with minimal cathexis is far more efficient; the added activity in the form of conscious attention to the muscular behavior markedly reduces the efficiency, in this case the automatic fluency of speech. In the functional regression to the pretraumatic state, i.e., the earlier learning phase, both conscious imitative speech elements as well as, to a lesser degree, the still earlier unconscious or id lalling speech elements re-emerge. Together they do not totally replace the preconscious functioning with its characteristic fluency and feeling of confidence in its automaticity, but they burden the performance and—what is even more damaging—they seriously impair the feeling of self-confidence.

The greater activity and cathexis constitute the defensive reaction to the trauma. The speech behavior here is spastic. The aim is to approach the object again; it is counterphobic. But the symptom also contains expressions whose aim is flight, a phobic reaction. The speech behavior here shows evidence of decathexis—on the mental side momentary amnesias, and on the physical side ineffectual iterations. The speech flow is not effectively propelled.

Two remote and major consequences result from this pathologic distortion of the ego automatism of speech when it becomes chronic. One is that (global) conception of verbalization in all that it encompasses is altered; the other is a significant deviation of the personality. The two are interrelated and will be treated in close order.

The speech function involves an address, an addressee, an act or a product—verbalization—and an aim: communication. As is well known, when the speech function is fully developed, each one of these elements is predominantly under the control of the secondary process. That is, while the primordial drive energies cathect the function, they do so in a state of dialectic fusion and are oriented realistically. The function itself becomes freed of id attributes; it becomes autonomous. Like a good mirror, it conveys the message with a minimal intrusion of itself. Magical concepts of self and object hallucinatory percepts of sounds, and instinctualized qualities of phonation and articulation stemming from early phases of ego and drive development have been outlived or adequately repressed. Trauma, on the other hand, affects each one of these component elements, partly through regression and partly through new pathological formations.

As was already mentioned with respect to the drives, splitting is a major consequence and characteristic. The addresser, the self, is split into two self-representations. The one representation, that of a stutterer, is regarded as damaged, not merely partially but in a total sense, and not merely functionally but more or less organically as well. The other, the compensatory self, more deeply repressed, is that of a great Demosthenes-like orator. It is as if the pluses and minuses of the function, and now the total personality identified with it, have been split asunder, defused, and polarized. The first is a denigrated image cathected by aggressive energy. It must not be exposed, but it is revealed by projection onto the addressee. He is feared as one who is aggressive and aims to humiliate the addresser. The second image is an idealized and libidinized one which craves adulation, to be noticed to be applauded.

The addressee is conceived as the ideal self—complete, "whole cloth." The attitudes toward him include envy, hostility, fear, a wish to humiliate and to reverse the roles. But the addresser also has reactive attitudes of guilt and masochistic submission. The speech function, now experienced as a symptom, becomes involved in conveying this multitude of attitudes and affects. It comes to serve exhibitionistic and perfectionistic aims simultaneously with masochistic, placating aims. The symptom, furthermore, being a vehicle in object relations, becomes a fixed reservoir of energy or raw material, which lends itself as a vehicle for expression of other complexes, such as the classical neurotic preoedipal and oedipal castration, and conflicts from practically all the instinctual levels. It must be emphasized, however, that these are later secondary and tertiary accretions. The total speech disorder is more than a neurotic conflict over the content of the message. Its taproot is an altered function of an automatic instrument with a subsequent altered concept of the act of verbalization and its participants. This alteration began in an early cumulative series of traumatic events involving self-differentiation at a time when speech was evolving from its archaic meanings.

One other attribute attesting to the archaic foundation of the symptom has been suggested before. It is the paranoid attitude toward nonstutterers. Its quality resembles that described by Hitschmann (1912) as pseudoparanoid, wherein the alloplastic elements are lacking and only the autoplastic character is prominent. The lack of self-differentiation accounts for this paranoid feature which brings stuttering close to the phenomenon of magical gestures in which nonverbal communication contains references to both addresser and addressee. Another similarly archaic phenomenon is Winnicott's concept of a transitional object (1953) in the sense of a creative expression which unites in itself both subject and object.

Perhaps it would be useful for this and other examples of disturbed ego automatisms to dispense with the term symptom, however useful it may be descriptively, for it does not meet the rigorous definition of the classical neurotic symptom as an attempted compromise between instinct and defense. As a matter of fact, an early nosological classification in child psychiatry referred to stuttering as a "trait" rather than a symptom, probably suggesting a not quite fully developed pathologic entity.

When I think of resemblances to disturbed ego automatisms

there comes to my mind the *actual neurosis* (Freud, 1895). This is another archaic disturbance, traumatic-phobic in nature, involving an alteration in physical functioning, due, I believe, to an alteration in cathexis, and resembling an intoxication, and finally serving as the base or nucleus for the fully developed neurosis with which it merges.

The distortion of the product, verbalization, and its aim, communication, can be described jointly. We can sense here the affects engendered during the initial traumatic interruptions in the learning experience. The interruption was sensed preconsciously as a separation and as a danger. Reactive hostility of the anal and oral modalities was liberated but repressed, and was experienced as anxiety within a social situation geared to communication. The unconscious hostility was merged with the stream of verbalization, both pushing for expression and relief of tension. There took place a condensation of speech and anal aggression with the aim of expression and separation (flight) and/or oral aggression. Thus the product, verbalization, was loaded by extra cathexis: unconscious hostility pressing for expression plus conscious anxiety. The latter, in turn, led to flight or decathexis. The aggression-loaded product was propelled toward the addressee as a forceful flow and approach, and away from the addressee as a withdrawal, or as a flow too weak to maintain itself. From now on the climate of any speech and social situation begins to be perceived as aggressivized, as was the verbalized message. The speech organ and function itself is unconsciously regarded as damaged.

These consequences of trauma are accompanied by libidinization of the injured function. There is first a mobilization of narcissistic libido cathecting the function (compensatory overevaluation); later on there emerge passive wishes for further investment with libido from objects, the so-called Demosthenes image of the speech and the compulsive need for exhibiting it. In addition, because both these aspects are associated with anxiety, there ensues a defensive increase of conscious attention. This plus the burden of increased preconscious cathexis turns the automatism into a state of *dysautomatization*.

In these patients the speech symptom is the most dramatic one, but this is not a monosymptomatic disorder. There are also less dramatic disturbances in other automatisms of muscular coordination and mental functioning—a general tendency to hesitation, blocking, and dysrhythmia. In time, the stutter and these other manifestations come to serve, as mentioned before, in the manner of the *actual neurotic* core of a neurosis, as the nucleus of an overlaying, more or less *specific characterology*. I will refer to the latter and its rather unique relation to the symptom after I deal with some additional functions affected by dysautomatization.

I have presented a composite of the main elements in the dysautomatization syndrome, some of its principal genetic elements, and a few characterological sequelae. Some illustrative clinical examples will clarify the picture. A young woman of 26 who stuttered showed many evidences of the trauma of separation. Throughout the life of the patient, her mother was partially invalided by various physical complaints based on an underlying mental illness. The patient was impressed that beneath the facade of pleasure in mothering, her mother was burdened by the responsibility. The stutter began shortly after her mother collapsed into helpless inactivity during a vacation trip and had to be hospitalized. The symptom was aggravated on all occasions of change denoting separation, such as moving to a new house, a new school, or taking a trip. Her life was filled with obsessive repetitions of the memory of her mother's breakdown, of anticipations of her own death, of the death of her parents and of her sister. Traumatic memories possessed a heightened degree of clarity; the same was true of her consciousness of self in almost all of its aspects and the most varied circumstances. The feeling was associated with ideas of separateness, unattractiveness, and inability to cope with almost all the details of daily living to the point of wondering how she could get through the day "in one piece"—all this despite steady, productive, intellectual activity of a high order. She was surprised at and did not believe the praise she received for her work as a teacher of advanced studies. The great effort she put out, and her actual misconception of an accentuated feeling of the difficulty of most of her tasks, was due to her mistrust of her automatic functions, including her memory. Instead, she leaned on over-alert conscious perceptions, especially self-perceptions. Her sense of ego weakness was composed of her lack of confidence in her preconscious functioning and its decathexis in favor of conscious hypercathexis, in itself a less economic and obviously more fatiguing modality. Her sharply focused attention to whatever she attempted to do, i.e., her trying to live through an exaggerated dependence on her conscious ego functions, was best portrayed in her sleep and sexual functions. She had difficulty in falling asleep, slept lightly, and was easily wakened; hence was inadequately refreshed on waking. Obviously, she could not allow herself easily to decathect what she relied on most, her conscious ego. Similarly, while she enjoyed intercourse she could not allow herself to reach orgasm, another expression of relinquishment of conscious ego control, in favor of what is more like a preconscious automatism. Her associations to this difficulty revealed the related phenomenon of fear of separation following orgasm and the wish to prolong indefinitely the sense of symbolic (i.e., maternal transference) closeness derived from the coital act.

This patient also suffered from anorexia nervosa. A major determinant of this symptom was the tense and anxious moments at mealtimes in her childhood, her mother overburdened and her father overcritical and examining the food as if it were poison. These experiences aggravated the separation anxiety with a heightened sense of oral aggression. Eating became an unpleasant, laborious act. The resultant suppression of hunger was probably due either to a suppression of the gastric musculosecretory activities which determine hunger or to repression of awareness of them. What this symptom had in common with the others is the disturbance in the rhythm of a somatopsychic automatism conditioned by a traumatizing milieu, even though the function involved a viscus of nonstriated muscle, and the disturbance in the automatism was expressed physically as an inhibition.

So far I have stressed the function of speech as it is affected by dysautomatization together with a group of other functions, such as locomotion and respiration, in which the component of muscular activity is prominent. The activity affected most commonly is the fluency of articulation in the form of iteration, prolongation, blocking. Sound production, or phonation as such, is seldom or only secondarily influenced, and is then not grossly noticeable. However, *vocalized* articulated speech is only the final link in a chain of elements constituting the act of verbalization. Immediately antecedent to verbalization is inner, silent speech that flows imperceptibly out of the complex process of thinking. We know that the important operational links of perception, memory and recall, monitoring and feedback, to mention only some of them, function predominantly preconsciously.

There is evidence too that the preverbalization phases of the stuttering patient are not infrequently affected by a similar flight of preconscious cathexis as in the case of the speech function. I have observed fleeting amnesias in the substance of the thinking process as distinct from blocks or verbal elements held firmly in the conscious mind. Others have reported lapses in the auditory feedback of the verbalization. Contractions in the size of the mental image of self and object with associated distortion of the sense of distance reported to me are, on the other hand, manifestations of cathectic change in the total setting of communcations involving the addresser and addressee. What all these phenomena have in common is a quality, the experience of a feeling of depersonalization or derealization. This is explicable as a flight of the normal cathexis of the particular part-function, with a resultant libidinal decathexis, and the emergence of an altered cathectic distribution containing a large quantity of free-floating aggression. Both the flight of the normal cathexis and the advent of the altered state account for the disorganized functioning and the feeling of strangeness or depersonalization.

Incidentally, though this subject deserves separate and fuller treatment, I cannot refrain from stating here a long-held conviction that depersonalization is the core symptom of the actual neurosis. All the actual neuroses I have observed contain a disturbance of function of automatic rhythm, a change of quality of cathexis and depersonalization. The depersonalized feeling and behavior are in my view similar or analogous to an intoxication. They are not a true intoxication but an alteration of cathexis. It is generally thought that Freud believed that the actual neurosis results from some chemical change in the sexual hormones whereas in fact he equivocated on this matter. In some passages he did state that the actual neurosis represents a chemical alteration; in others, that the behaviour *resembles* an intoxication, for example, thyrotoxicosis. I incline toward the second possibility. A recent survey by a neuro-logist examining a group of men suspected of driving in a state of alcoholic intoxication showing some muscular incoordination re-vealed a substantial number of neurologic and other metabolic disturbances which have a superficial resemblance to alcoholic intoxication but were not due to it. Emotional disturbances were not listed and were probably not looked for.

Augusta Bonnard (see Kavka, 1962, pp. 174–176), writing on impediments of speech, focused on what she called the dys-synergic muscular mechanisms with special reference to the tongue. She described the defense reaction to trauma as "defensive mimic-ry" of the aggressor by means of ticlike tongue movements which she regards as a form of true conversion which thereafter merges with an innate, non-visual, subliminal order of lingual cathexis. It seems to me that a merging of such disparate muscular rhythm patterns pointing in opposite directions can account for the postu-lated dys-synergy. This view appears to approximate my own view on dysautomatization, though formulated in somewhat different terms. However, it is noteworthy that several discussants, Gitelson, Kohut, and others, associating some of their own experiences to Bonnard's presentation, stressed the aspect of depersonalization.

Maxwell Gitelson, in the same discussion, impressed by the clinical examples in the use of the tongue as an "alter-ego," was reminded of a patient who sometimes regarded his tongue as foreign to the ego. Since sensation and affects relating to the tongue were dissociated or isolated, what seemed to be operating could be called depersonalization in respect to the tongue. Perhaps the term "motoric depersonalization" aptly describes some of the phe-nomena observed in Dr. Bonnard's patients.

Heinz Kohut's comment was almost identical with my formu-lation. He concluded that the tongue of a three-and-a-half-year-old boy with a temporary stammer was "estranged from the child's ego"—i.e., depersonalized. His lucid description of the ego split I referred to above warrants citation. He observed the boy indirectly through the analysis of his father. This patient's personality was blurred and he often reacted to his own perverse transgressions by becoming harshly critical toward his son. Dr. Kohut speculated that such criticism (which is not related to the child's impulses but is due to the child's inclusion into the narcissistic system of the educator) cannot become part of the child's superego; instead, there is fixation on a more primitive phase of drive control through a narcissistically experienced "object." No object-directed rebellion against the father (or against the superego) is possible. The tongue becomes the battleground of pre-verbal rage, in the service of a rebellion that has no differentiated object, and is thus estranged from the child's ego. The success of Dr. Bonnard's therapeutic efforts may be partly due to the fact that her attention to the child's tongue movements helps him to establish ownership and mastery of this organ.

At this point it may be well to discuss how to place or orient this disorder of dysautomatization in the general scheme of psycho-pathologic formation. What I will state refers mainly to the disorders of speech whose prototype is stuttering. I feel less certain about how to place the group of learning disorders based on deviations of perception and memory. These intellectual difficulties begin to be noticed at a later age than the speech symptoms; but the actual beginnings of the speech symptoms could be traced to an earlier age. I have classified these speech disorders along the line of the developmental phases of the ego before verbalization has fully developed and before self-differentiation has been completed. It is a functional deviation resulting from a fixation (before the learning phase has been completed) on a trauma and/or the defense against it.

Kohut states that "estrangement (of the tongue) from the child's ego . . ." represents a "*fixation* on a more *primitive* phase of drive control through a narcissistically experienced "object." It was Robert Gronner's impression, in the same discussion, that "a pathological defense mechanism similar to, yet distinct from intro-jection, in the sense of being archaic" was operative in Dr. Bonnard's cases.

It remains now to deal with the remote results of the trauma on (1) the further development of the "symptom," and on (2) the further development of the character of the patient. Regarding the first, the quotation marks around the term "symptom" are intended to point up the differences between this type of psychopathologic formation and the classical psychoneurotic symptom. Clinically, the stutter as a prototype starts some time after speech has already been established—about the third or fourth year. A peak time is the fifth or sixth year—corresponding to the more advanced stages of the speech development, also corresponding with the time of beginning of school as well as the height of the oedipal phase. At this time the stutter constitutes one of the most spontaneously resolvable of all symptoms. However, when it is not resolved at this time spontaneously or therapeutically, it continues to develop, and becomes rooted with characterologic concomitants right on through the latency period and adolescence. The psychoneurotic symptom, with the exception of some compulsive symptoms, does not usually emerge during latency but is delayed until adolescence. Again, unlike the psychoneurotic symptom, and in contrast to the relatively easy and frequent resolution shortly after onset, the stutter of the adult is among the most refractory of symptoms.

Classical psychoanalysis may lessen the severity of the stuttering symptom, but seldom, if ever, effects a complete resolution. The syndrome operates on two levels which are not confluent but isolated. Much in the character structure insofar as it is of the neurotic type, can be influenced by psychoanalysis. To the extent that the symptom reflects that type of character, it is resolved with the latter. However, to the extent that the symptom is related to the nuclear fixation on the original trauma and its defense—a fixation which is isolated from the neurotic character structure and apparently cannot be dealt with by the classical analytic technique—it remains uninfluenced.

A major difficulty in dealing with the stutter is that it is a disturbance of an automatism serving an important adaptation. Because of this, even though the general increased consciousness and attention cathexes plus some id elements burden the functioning, the stutter itself partakes in the adaptative functioning and becomes secondarily libidinized and automatized. It becomes ego-syntonic. Thus the patient is not always fully conscious of it and he offers resistance to the therapist's efforts to make it conscious to him. He does not complain of it. To make the stutter ego-dystonic by analyzing its analogues in other areas, the purpose it serves, and at what price, to make again conscious his adaptation which has become automatized, requires a degree of focusing on the symptom and a degree of activity customarily not regarded as proper analytic technique. The tenacity of the symptom and its use or adaptation also stem from the fixed idea of the damaged self-image, and hatred of it, both of which are projected outward. The tenacity of those fixed ideas often approximates the tenacity of delusions.

It is no wonder that at this point of *impasse* in treatment it is a common practice among analysts to send the "intractable patient" to a speech therapist because the stutter is "now a habit." The speech therapist does not work with the ambivalences; and he is sometimes more successful, especially if the patient does not come in order to prove his "intractability" to his family and therapist. Occasionally the patient comes to me at this point. I found that the stutter per se cannot be touched before much energy has been spent on working through the ambivalence and the resistance. When the patient reaches a plateau of predominant positive transference, it is then possible to work through the "gains" as well as the price he pays characterologically (i.e., analogically and away from the symptom) for these "gains." This work is essential for the motivation in therapy. Some of the rock-bottom phenomena here, such as the idea of a damaged organ and organism, and the most welcome use of the symptom as an "indispensable" crutch, have attained psychotic-like tenacity. To relinquish these—his own highly cathected, uniquely functioning maladaptations and to cathect a "foreign" adaptation, fluent speech—amounts to a new learning situation. To the extent that it can approximate or simulate the original, normal speech-learning situation, a consistent unambivalent milieu, a recathexis of an unwatched, preconscious automatism can evolve and take the place of the pathological one. The process brings to mind that of an organ transplant, even though these patients have experienced an early period as well as intercurrent periods of fluent speech. When it is attained it is a triumph of the establishment of a consistent positive identification over a tenacious ambivalent one that dominated the self for many years.

We come now to the final point, the character structure that constitutes the organization of the distant sequelae of the dysautomatization. This large subject can be dealt with here only in outline form. The severity of deviation depends on quantitative factors and the duration. Perhaps those factors account for the different experiences and different conceptual emphases of different authors.

In the symptom, I have stressed the consciousness of damage felt by the patient in regard to his speech function and the resultant increased watchfulness and control of it. These reactions, enlarged and elaborated, are reflected within the personality as heightened total self-consciousness, and constitute its central fixation. In the course of development other conflicts, including the classical neurotic ones, are attracted to this fixation. Disguising their identity, they express themselves through the speech symptom. The disorder thus becomes overdetermined and is frequently experienced as a monosymptomatic one. The subjective self-image is usally one of a part-object, and is regarded with shame. The attitude toward objects is passive and aggressive, with a feeling of being persecuted, in the sense of being ridiculed, by these supposedly complete individuals. The true self and its potentials are prevented from experiencing and reacting to life spontaneously because it is blocked by the constant interactions between the false self-image and its compensations and the false image of objects. Speech and social situations become perverted into instruments of and settings for aggression and appeasement. Due to ambivalence and oscillation between flight and approach, hesitation in action is marked in the character as disturbed fluency is in the symptom. These individuals frequently show other dysfluencies in writing, playing the piano, walking, and driving. Parallel disturbances in the partial automatisms of mental functioning are reflected in transient amnesias and perceptive deficiencies.

I wish now to mention a few excerpts from the literature referring to stuttering per se or linked as part of a group of similar disorders. I find the similarities and contrasts with my views instructive. As a point of departure, I will recapitulate my view that stuttering, per se, (and as prototype?) is a twofold disorder. It is first a symptom in the sense of a fixation or a traumatic disturbance of the rhythm of a psychosomatic automatism, as well as a fixation on the defense which also contributes to the rhythm disturbance, both during the advanced learning phase of the function. Secondarily, later conflicts of the classical neuroses make use of this fixation in the automatism. This fixation determines a special type of super-imposed character disorder which in general reflects the structure of the symptom. The symptom, and in part the character, cannot be explicated in terms of the classical neurotic symptom. Rather it can be in special terms—that of a trauma affecting an automatism producing a fixation on it and on its defense.

Bonnard, as reported by Kavka (1962), said that she "found the ego development of children with speech impediments to be normal or even greater than normal in strength and precocity." This is most likely the group I mentioned above which has a large percentage of spontaneous resolution. She added that, "while their disability tends to debar them from attaining their potential stations in life, they are usually worthwhile personalities as is shown in situations requiring courage or tenacity of purpose" (p. 174). While I would not question their worthwhileness as personalities, in my experience what debars them from attaining their potential stations in life is not their symptomatic disability per se but the associated character structure.

Dosuzkov (1965) of Prague regards stuttering as belonging to what he calls the fourth transference neurosis, a clinical entity he terms skoptophobia:

> The main symptom of skoptophobia is fear of public exposure and disgrace, a belittling associated with convictions of physical or mental inferiority. The syndrome of skoptophobia has the following charac-teristics: the fear of public exposure or disgrace, inferiority feelings; pathoaidoia (sense of shame of one's own disorder); ideas about relationships which lead to fear of objects and which can culminate in ostracism, and manifestations of pathological shyness. An extraordi-narily strong sense of shame is a characteristic sign of this neurosis, as anxiety is the main feature of anxiety hysteria, and compulsion of compulsion neurosis. This sense of shame is at the base of skopto-phobia and thereby distinguishes it from hysterical phobias based on anxiety, as well as from compulsion neuroses based on unconscious aggression.
>
> . . . The course is chronic, with occasional remissions. It begins in the second half of childhood following a preceding hysteria, enuresis or compulsion neurosis. It leads to an impressive shyness and to other attempts to hide the sense of shame which may reach the height of complete rejection of interpersonal relations. Some cases occasionally

end up with termination of social contacts, designated above as ostracism. The pathological ideas about interpersonal relations may reach psychotic proportions. . . . the skoptophobic avoids social contacts out of fear that the environment will ridicule him; he is anxious about the environmental aggression; the compulsive neurotic fears his own aggression. . . . The instinctual fixation among skoptophobics is on the sadistic impulses, generally on the anal, urethral, and exhibitionistic, less often oral components.

The uniqueness of the stuttering symptom as a disturbance of an automatism, its relative separateness from the associated characterological disorder, unlike the greater fusion of the two in the classical neuroses—the point of view developed in this paper—is not shared by most authors in its entirety, though it is corroborated in a number of distinct aspects, notably in Dosuzkov's formulation.

Summary

Speech is viewed as the prototype of a group of complex ego functions that operate automatically, i.e., preconsciously. Stuttering is conceptualized as the prototype of dysautomatization, a trauma-induced disturbance that is frequently a transitory symptom. If it persists into latency and adolescence, it becomes a chronic syndrome that has two major aspects: the primary disturbance is the stutter as a symptom, a fixation resulting from early trauma; secondarily, later neurotic conflicts are engrafted upon and utilize the primary fixation. Moreover, the fixation determines the development of a character disorder which in general tends to reflect the structure of the fixation. Classical psychoanalytic technique may succeed in resolving the neurotic elements. Successful treatment of the primary fixation requires reeducational methods. The clinical and theoretical considerations are illustrated by the case of an adult female stutterer.

Additional Reading

1. I. Peter Glauber. Further contributions to the concept of stuttering. *Journal of the Hillside Hospital,* 1962, 11(4).

2. W. Clifford M. Scott. Finger-licking finger-flicking habit. *Journal of the American Psychoanalytic Association*, 1963, 11:832–834.

3. E. Weiss. *The Structure and Dynamics of the Human Mind.* New York: Grune & Stratton, 1960. (See material on depersonalization)

4. S. Freud. An autobiographical study, *Standard Edition*, 1925, 20:25–26.

5. _____. Fragments of an analysis of a case of hysteria, p. 113; Three essays on the theory of sexuality, pp. 215–216; My views on the part played by sexuality in the etiology of the neuroses, p. 279; Psychical (all mental) treatment, p. 284. All in *Standard Edition*, 1905, 7.

References

Abraham, K. (1916) The first pregenital stage of the libido. In *Selected Papers on Psychoanalysis*. New York: Brunner/Mazel, 1979, pp. 248–279.

———— (1924) A short study of the development of the libido, viewed in the light of mental disorders. In *Selected Papers on Psychoanalysis*. New York: Brunner/Mazel, 1979, pp. 418–501.

Balkanyi, C. (1961) Psycho-analysis of a stammering girl. *International Journal of Psycho-Analysis*, 42:97–109.

Bergler, E. (1945) Thirty-some years after Ferenczi's "Stages in the development of the sense of reality." *Psychoanalytic Review*, 32:125–145, No. 2.

Bergmann, M. (1963) The place of Federn's ego psychology in psychoanalytic metapsychology. *Journal of the American Psychoanalytic Association*, 11:97–116.

Blanton, S. (1956) Unpublished discussion. Recorded in the Archives of the A. A. Brill Library of the New York Psychoanalytic Society.

Blum, E. (1926) The psychology of study and examinations. *International Journal of Psycho-Analysis*, 7:457–469.

Breuer, J., and Freud, S. (1893–1895) Studies on hysteria. *Standard Edition*,* 2:45–105; 135–181.

Brill, A. A. (1923) Speech disturbances in nervous and mental diseases. *Quarterly Journal of Speech Education*, 9:129–135.

———— (1941) Necrophilia. *Journal of Criminal Psychopathology*, 2:433–443; 3:51–73.

Bunker, H. A. (1934) The voice as (female) phallus. *Psychoanalytic Quarterly*, 3:391–429.

Bychowski, G. (1945) The ego of homosexuals. *International Journal of Psycho-Analysis*, 26:114–127.

---

*Unless otherwise indicated, all references to Freud's writings are to the *Standard Edition of the Complete Psychological Works of Sigmund Freud*, 24 Vols., translated and edited by James Strachey. New York: Norton.

170

Coriat, I. H. (1928) *Stammering: A Psychoanalytic Interpretation.* New York/ Washington, D.C.: Nervous and Mental Disease Monograph Publishing Company.

―――― (1933) The dynamics of stammering. *Psychoanalytic Quarterly,* 2:244–259.

―――― (1943) The psychoanalytic concept of stammering. *The Nervous Child,* 2:167–171.

Deri, Frances (1942) Neurotic disturbances of sleep: A symposium. *International Journal of Psycho-Analysis,* 23:56–59.

Dosuzkov, T. (1965) Skoptophobia―die vierte Übertragungsneurose. *Psyche,* 19:537–546.

Eisenson, J. (1958) Causes of stuttering. Unpublished manuscript, Queens College, New York.

Federn, P. (1952) Narcissism in the structure of the ego. *Ego Psychology and the Psychoses.* New York: Basic Books.

Fenichel, O. (1939) The counter-phobic attitude. *Collected Papers,* second series. New York: Norton, pp. 163–173.

―――― (1945) *The Psychoanalytic Theory of Neurosis.* New York: Norton, pp. 152–153.

Ferenczi, S. (1911) On obscene words. In *Contributions to Psychoanalysis.* New York: Basic Books/Brenner, 1950, pp. 132–153.

―――― (1913) Stages in the development of the sense of reality. In *Contributions to Psychoanalysis.* New York: Basic Books/Brenner, 1950, pp. 213–239.

―――― (1921) Psycho-analytic observations on tic. In *Further Contributions to Psychoanalysis.* New York: Basic Books, 1952, pp. 142–173.

―――― (1917) Disease- or patho-neuroses. In *Further Contributions to Psychoanalysis.* New York: Basic Books, 1952, pp. 78–88.

―――― (1928) Gulliver phantasies. In *Final Contributions to Psychoanalysis.* New York: Basic Books, 1955, pp. 41–60.

Freud, A. (1936) *The Ego and the Mechanisms of Defense.* New York: International Universities Press, 1966.

Freud, S. (1893) A case of successful treatment by hypnotism. *Standard Edition,* 1:117–128.

―――― (1895) On the grounds for detaching a particular syndrome from neurasthenia under the description "anxiety neurosis." *Standard Edition,* 3:87–115.

―――― (1897-1902) *Origins of Psycho-Analysis.* New York: Basic Books, 1954.

―――― (1898) Sexuality in the aetiology of the neuroses. *Standard Edition,* 3:261–285.

―――― (1901) The psychopathology of everyday life. *Standard Edition.*

―――― (1905) Three essays on the theory of sexuality. *Standard Edition,* 7:125–243.

―――― (1909) Five lectures on psycho-analysis. *Standard Edition,* 11:3–55.

―――― (1911a) Formulations regarding the two principles in mental functioning. *Standard Edition,* 12:215–226.

_____ (1911b) Psycho-analytic notes upon an autobiographical account of a case of paranoia (Dementia Paranoides). *Standard Edition*, 2:3–82.

_____ (1912) Recommendations to physicians practicing psycho-analysis. *Standard Edition*, 12:109–120.

_____ (1913) The disposition to obsessional neurosis. *Standard Edition*, 12:313–326.

_____ (1914) On narcissism. *Standard Edition*, 14:69–102.

_____ (1915) The unconscious. *Standard Edition*, 14:161–215.

_____ (1916) Some character types met with in psycho-analytic work. *Standard Edition*, 14:311–333.

_____ (1920a) Beyond the pleasure principle. *Standard Edition*, 18:3–64.

_____ (1920b) The psychogenesis of a case of homosexuality in a woman. *Standard Edition*, 18:146–172.

_____ (1922) Some neurotic mechanisms in jealousy, paranoia and homosexuality. *Standard Edition*, 18:222–232.

_____ (1923) The ego and the id. *Standard Edition*, 19:3–66.

_____ (1924) The economic problem of masochism. *Standard Edition*, 19:157–170.

_____ (1926) Inhibitions, symptoms and anxiety. *Standard Edition*, 20:77–174. Also: *The Problem of Anxiety*. H. A. Bunker, trans. New York: Norton, 1936.

_____ (1927) Postscript to a discussion on lay analysis. *Standard Edition*, 20:251–258.

_____ (1937) Analysis terminable and interminable. *Standard Edition*, 23:211–253.

_____ (1939) Moses and monotheism. *Standard Edition*, 23:3–137.

Gerard, M. (1947) The psychogenic tic in ego development. *The Psychoanalytic Study of the Child*, 2:133–162. New York: International Universities Press.

Glauber, I. P. (1935) The treatment of the functional speech disorders in a medical-social clinic: Implications for the treatment of functional disorders in general. *American Journal of Orthopsychiatry*.

_____ (1943) Psychoanalytic concepts of the stutterer. *Nervous Child*.

_____ (1944) Speech characteristics of psychoneurotic patients. *Journal of Speech Disorders*.

_____ (1944) A social-psychiatric therapy for the stutterer. *Newsletter of American Association of Psychiatric Social Workers*.

_____ (1949) Observations on a primary form of anhedonia. *Psychoanalytic Quarterly*.

_____ (1950) The nature and treatment of stuttering. *Social Casework*.

_____ (1950a) Ego development and the character of the stutterer. Abstract by Charles Brenner in *Psychoanalytic Quarterly*.

_____ (1951) The mother in the etiology of stuttering. Abstract by Sidney Tarchow in *Psychoanalytic Quarterly*.

_____ (1952) Dynamic therapy for the stutterer. *Specialized Techniques in Psychotherapy*. New York: Basic Books.

_____ (1953) A deterrent in the study and practice of medicine. *Psychoanalytic Quarterly*.

_____ (1955) On the meaning of agoraphilia. *Journal of the American Psychoanalytic Association*.

_____ (1956) The rebirth motif in homosexuality and its teleological significance. *International Journal of Psycho-Analysis*.

_____ (1958) The psychoanalysis of stuttering. In *Stuttering: A Symposium*. New York: Harper and Row.

_____ (1958a) Freud's contribution on stuttering: Their relation to some current insights. *Journal of the American Psychoanalytic Association*.

_____ (1959) Notes on the early stages in the development of stuttering. *Journal of the Hillside Hospital*.

_____ (1962) Further contributions to the concept of stuttering. *Journal of the Hillside Hospital*.

_____ (1963) Federn's annotation of Freud's theory of anxiety. *Journal of the American Psychoanalytic Association*.

_____ (1966) Discussion of "The Psychodynamic Formulation of Agoraphobia" by E. Weiss in *Forum*.

_____ (1968) Dysautomatization: a disorder of preconscious ego functioning. *The International Journal of Psycho-Analysis*, Part 1, 1968.

Glover, E. (1927) Lectures on techniques in psycho-analysis. *International Journal of Psycho-Analysis*, 8:486–520.

_____ (1939) *Psycho-Analysis*. London: Staples.

Greenacre, P. (1952) *Trauma, Growth, and Personality*, Chapter 14. New York: International Universities Press.

Grinker, R., and Spiegel, J. (1945) *War Neuroses*. Philadelphia: Blakiston.

Hahn, E. (1943) *Stuttering: Significant Theories and Therapies*. Stanford, Calif.: Stanford University Press.

Hartmann, H. (1939) *Ego Psychology and the Problem of Adaptation*. New York: International Universities Press, 1958.

_____ (1950) Comments on the psychoanalytic theory of the ego. In *Essays on Ego Psychology*. New York: International Universities Press, 1964, pp. 113–141.

_____, Kris, E., and Loewenstein, R. (1946) Comments on the formation of pschic structure. *The Psychoanalytic Study of the Child*, 2:11–38. New York: International Universities Press.

Hitschmann, E. (1912) Swedenborg's paranoia. *Yearbook of Psychoanalysis*, 6:281–285. New York: International Universities Press, 1950.

Hoffer, W. (1949) Mouth, hand and ego integration. *The Psychoanalytic Study of the Child*, 3/4:49–56. New York: International Universities Press.

Jackson, H. (1878) On affections of speech from disease of the brain. *Brain*, 1:304.

Jacobson, E. (1943) Depression: The Oedipus conflict in the development of depressive mechanisms. *Psychoanalytic Quarterly*, 12:541–556.

――― (1953) Contribution to the metapsychology of cyclothymic depression. In P. Greenacre, ed., *Affective Disorders*, New York: International Universities Press, pp. 49–83.

Jespersen, O. (1922) *Language: Its Nature, Development and Origin.* London: Allen and Unwin.

Jones, E. (1911) Psychopathology of everyday life. In *Papers in Psycho-Analysis*, 4th ed. Baltimore: William Wood, 1938, pp 56–119.

――― (1955) *The Life and Work of Sigmund Freud,* 2:183. New York: Basic Books.

Karlin, I. (1947) Psychosomatic theory of stuttering. *Journal of Speech and Hearing Disorders*, 12:319–322.

Katan, A. (1951) The role of displacement in agoraphobia. *International Journal of Psycho-Analysis*, 32:41–51.

Kavka, J., Reporter (1962) Impediments of speech; a special psychosomatic instance, by A. Bonnard. *Bulletin of the Philadelphia Association for Psychoanalysis*, 12:174–176.

Kempner, S. (1925) Some remarks on oral erotism. *International Journal of Psycho-Analysis*, 6:419–429.

Kris, E. (1950) On preconscious mental processes. In *Psychoanalytic Explorations in Art*. New York: International Universities Press, 1952, pp. 303–320.

Laufer, M., Dinhoff, E., and Solomons, G. (1957) Hyperkinetic impulse disorders in children's behavior problems. *Psychosomatic medicine*, 19:38–49.

Lewin, B. D. (1933) The body as phallus. In *Selected Writings*. New York: The Psychoanalytic Quarterly, Inc., 1973, pp. 28–47.

――― (1935) Claustrophobia. In *Selected Writings*. New York: The Psychoanalytic Quarterly, Inc., 1973, pp. 48–54.

――― (1946a) Countertransferences in the technique of medical practice. In *Selected Writings*. New York: The Psychoanalytic Quarterly, Inc. 1973, pp. 449–458.

――― (1946b) Sleep, the mouth, and the dream screen. In *Selected Writings*. New York: The Psychoanalytic Quarterly, Inc., 1973, pp. 87–100.

――― (1950) *The Psychoanalysis of Elation*. New York: Norton.

――― (1952) Phobic symptoms and dream interpretation. In *Selected Writings*. New York: The Psychoanalytic Quarterly, Inc., 1973, pp. 187–212.

Lieberman, H. (1924) Mono-symptomatic neuroses. *International Journal of Psycho-Analysis*, 5:393–394.

Nunberg, H. (1926) The sense of guilt and the need for punishment. In *The Practice and Theory of Psychoanalysis*. New York: International Universities Press, 1961, pp. 81–101.

———— (1931) Symbiotic function of the ego. In *The Practice and Theory of Psychoanalysis.* New York: International Universities Press, 1961, pp. 120–136.

———— (1938a) Homosexuality, magic and aggression. In *The Practice and Theory of Psychoanalysis.* New York: International Universities Press, 1961, pp. 150–164.

———— (1938b) Psychological interrelations between physician and patient. In *The Practice and Theory of Psychoanalysis.* New York: International Universities Press, 1961, pp. 174–184.

———— (1947) Circumcision and problems of bisexuality. *International Journal of Psycho-Analysis,* 28:145–179.

————, and Federn, E. (1975) *Minutes of the Vienna Psychoanalytic Society,* IV, 1912–1928. New York: International Universities Press.

Orton, S. (1928) Physiological theory of reading disability and stuttering in children. *New England Journal of Medicine,* 199:1046.

Parson, B. (1924) *Left-Handedness.* New York: Macmillan.

Reich, W. (1933) *Character Analysis.* New York: Farrar, Straus and Giroux, 1972.

Ribble, M. (1941) Disorganizing factors of infant personality. *American Journal of Psychiatry,* 98:459–463.

Ribot, T. (1897) *The Psychology of the Emotions.* London: W. Scott.

Róheim, G. (1945) *War, Crime and the Covenant.* Monticello, N.Y.: Medical Journal Press.

Schmideberg, M. (1930) The rise of psychotic mechanisms in cultural development. *International Journal of Psycho-Analysis,* 11:387–415.

———— (1942) Some observations on individual reactions to air raids. *International Journal of Psycho-Analysis,* 23:146–176.

Seemann, M. (1934) Über somatische Befunde bei Stotterern. *Monatsch. f. Ohrenh.* 68:895–914.

Segal, H. (1953) A necrophilic fantasy. *International Journal of Psycho-Analysis,* 34:98–102.

Simmel, E. (1926) The doctor-game illness and the profession of medicine. *International Journal of Psycho-Analysis,* 7:470–483.

Slavson, S. (1943) *An Introduction to Group Therapy.* New York: The Commonwealth Fund.

Szondi, L. (1932) Konstitutionsanalyse von 100 Stotterern. *Wien. med. Wochenschrift,* 82:922–928.

Tausk, V. (1934) On the origin of the "infuencing machine" in schizophrenia. *Psychoanalytic Quarterly,* 3:391–429.

Waelder, R. (1929) Review of Freud's *Inhibitions, Symptom and Anxiety.* In *Psychoanalysis: Observation, Theory, Application.* New York: International Universities Press, 1976, pp. 57–67.

———— (1960). *Basic Theory of Psychoanalysis.* New York: International Universities Press.

Wassef, W. (1961) Etude clinique de différentes modalités structurales au cour de psychanalyse de bégues. *Rev. Franc. Psychanal.,* 19:440–473. Abstracted in *The Annual Survey of Psychoanalysis,* 6:157–160. New York: International Universities Press.

Weiss, E. (1952) Introduction to Paul Federn's *Ego Psychology and the Psychoses.* New York: Basic Books.

―――― (1960) *The Structure and Dynamics of the Human Mind.* New York: Grune & Stratton.

West, R. (1958) *Stuttering: A Symposium.* New York: Harper & Bros.

Winnicott, D. (1953) Transitional objects and transitional phenomena. In *Collected Papers.* New York: Basic Books, 1958, pp. 229–242.

Index